MW01366095

"This book is far more than just a resource of information to assist families impacted by any life altering illness; it's a story about humanity, from the doctor's offices to our most treasured caregiver. If we are brave enough to step 'outside the box,' there is hope!"

—D. Erickson, N.W. Wisconsin ALS Outreach Support Services

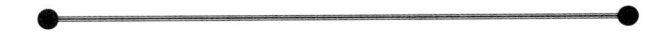

"After reading River of Hope I felt angry that the health care system is so unwilling to admit, let alone relinquish, the pieces it can't do... frustrated that we know so much about toxicities but are unwilling to consider the evidence that is there... thankful that David would share this story to help me find more energy and action to create the changes the health care system needs."

—Sue Peck, Nursing Professor and Nurse Practitioner

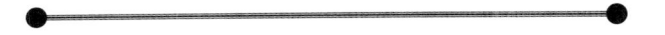

"Kathleen was a very special human being. Despite having a terrible disease she always smiled. I don't think I could ever be such an empowered person. And also, you David were an incredible partner for her, standing by her and doing all you could to help her throughout her whole illness. You were both a great inspiration to my staff and me."

—Robert S. Waters, M.D.

RIVER OF HOPE

My Journey with Kathy
in Search of Healing from Lou Gehrig's Disease

David Tank

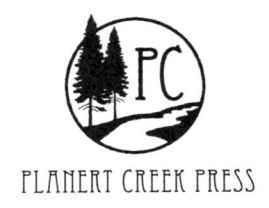

PLANERT CREEK PRESS

RIVER OF HOPE

My Journey with Kathy in Search of Healing from Lou Gehrig's Disease
by David Tank

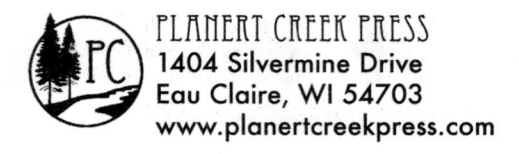

PLANERT CREEK PRESS
1404 Silvermine Drive
Eau Claire, WI 54703
www.planertcreekpress.com

Photos by David Tank and Kathy Tank

Copyright © 2008 by David Tank

ISBN 978-0-9815064-0-1

First Edition 2008

Printed and bound in the United States of America

Tank, David.
   My journey with Kathy : in search of healing from Lou Gehrig's disease / David Tank ; photos by David and Kathy Tank.
      p. cm.
   Summary: This true story chronicles the frustrations and joys of Kathy Tank as she fought to beat Lou Gehrig's disease (ALS). Kathy's story of determination and hope, her fight to beat a disease that the 'experts' told her was unbeatable, is both inspiring and tragic.
ISBN-13: 978-0-9815064-0-1
   1. Tank, Kathy–Biography. 2. Amyotrophic lateral sclerosis. 3. Amyotrophic lateral sclerosis–Patients–Biography. 4. Alternative medicine. 5. Medical personnel-caregiver relationships. I. Tank, Kathy. II. Title. III. Title: In search of healing from Lou Gehrig's disease.
   616.83
   362.1

                                                                           2008923303

"I decided last Sunday night on this move. I haven't been a bit of good to the team since the season started. It would not be fair to the boys, to [Coach] Joe (McCarthy) or to the baseball public for me to try going on. In fact, it would not be fair to myself, and I'm the last consideration.

"It's tough to see your mates on base, have a chance to win a ball game and not be able to do anything about it.

"Maybe a rest will do me some good. Maybe it won't. Who knows? Who can tell? *I'm just hoping.*"

—Lou Gehrig

Negotiating ALS is like running a wild river in a leaky kayak, without a paddle. You keep sinking lower and lower at the same time that you're being swept downstream, and you have no control over either one.

The medical experts stand watching on the riverbank, measuring how far you get and timing how long it takes you to hit bottom.

Wouldn't you rather have someone jump in with you, help you repair the leak, give you a paddle, and teach you how to negotiate your way out of the river? Or better yet, make sure that the kayak is sound and fully equipped before they let you begin your journey?

Thank you...

...to Michael Martin, Rob Reid, Ann Heywood, Julie Watts, Maryann Welker and Ron Tank for reading early manuscripts of this story and encouraging me to continue writing, and to Kyle Kingston for proofreading.

...to the kind and gentle people described on these pages who helped Kathy spend her life living instead of dying.

...and most of all, thank you to Kathy for being such an inspiration and model of courage, optimism and hope. I have no regrets.

CONTENTS

"Hope is imagining and fighting for what did not seem possible before."

—Barack Obama, 2/16/08
Eau Claire, Wisconsin

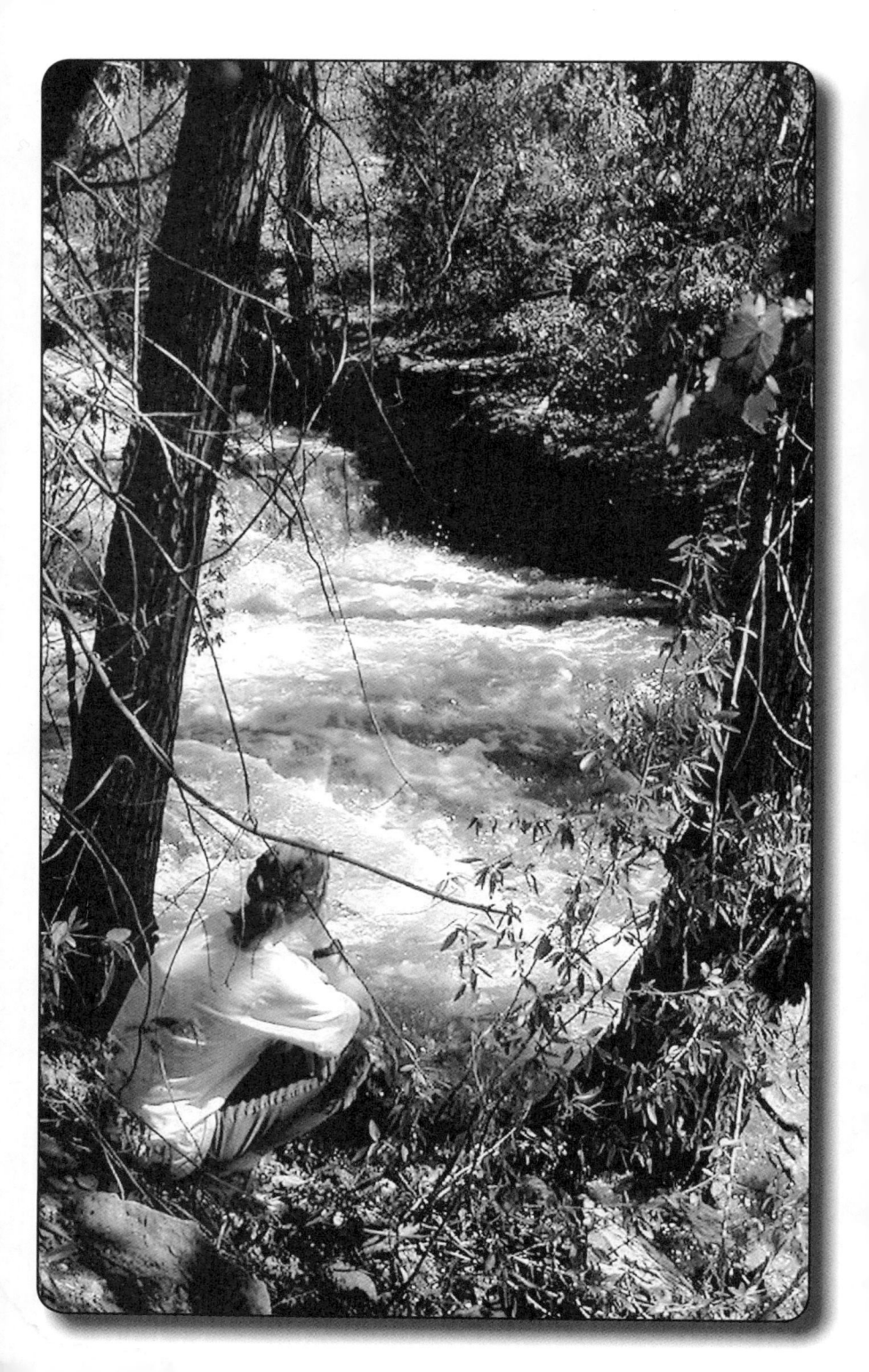

PROLOGUE
Why I am telling this story

When my wife, Kathy, was diagnosed with ALS in the spring of 2006, we were devastated. ALS, often called Lou Gehrig's disease, is a degenerative disorder that progressively destroys the nerves connecting your brain to your voluntary muscles. It is regularly described as being "rapidly progressive" and "invariably fatal," usually within a few years.

People with ALS often end up completely unable to move, trapped inside their own bodies while their minds stay fully functional. In the later stages of the disease, the person's only way to communicate may be with the blink of an eye or the twitch of a cheek muscle. While most cases of ALS begin in the legs and arms, Kathy's began in her throat and tongue, eliminating her ability to speak and swallow before it affected the other parts of her body.

The "experts" basically told us there was no hope. Instead of offering any suggestions to help Kathy get better, they advised us how to prepare for all of the awful things that lay ahead.

They showed us equipment that would help her breathe mechanically when she could no longer breathe on her own. They gave us literature about remodeling our home, so we'd be prepared when Kathy was strapped into a special wheelchair or trapped in her bed. They told us about organizations that may be able to help with some of the many expenses that we would be facing as the disease progressed.

None of it was *if.* All of it was *when.*

For many years, a highlight of Kathy's summers had been getting out and riding her bicycle. During the summer of 2005, the year before she was officially diagnosed with ALS (but was already in its early stages), she'd biked more than 3,000 miles.

Even though her legs were still strong in June 2006, the ALS specialists advised Kathy against much physical activity. They told her that it would only increase the progression of the disease, and that once the nerves to her muscles were gone the muscles would atrophy and there was no way that any of that could be reversed. It was as if they not only wanted to tell her about the horrible things that lay ahead, but also take away the enjoyable things that she could still do.

By mid summer of 2006, Kathy could barely swallow and had to have a feeding tube surgically placed into her abdomen. The surgery itself went fine, but incompetent nursing care during her stay in the hospital nearly killed her. When she came home, a health care specialist was there to teach us how to use the feeding tube. To our amazement, the health care "expert" had such limited knowledge of the subject that we ended up having to teach ourselves how to use it with regular food that we prepared on our own.

Hopeless. No other word better describes our feelings about the situation we were in.

Throughout the summer of 2006, Kathy faithfully took her prescribed medications, even though it seemed pointless. One drug, the only medication that was FDA approved for the treatment of ALS, had the potential of slowing the disease's progression by a whopping 60-90 days. The side effects were that it could, and did, increase Kathy's symptoms of her ALS.

Hopeless.

Another drug she was given was actually for an entirely different disease, but it was prescribed to her because of its side effect of causing severe dry mouth. The physician reasoned that it may help her with her drooling. It did. But combined with her other prescribed medications, it also essentially paralyzed her face, leaving her expressionless.

Hopeless.

Based on the information provided by the "experts," Kathy and I started planning how to enlarge the bedroom window, so that when she was unable to get out of bed or move her head, she could still watch the birds at the feeder.

We worried about how to deal with our tiny bathrooms, which were much too small to accommodate the wheelchair and other assistive devices that we were told she would soon be needing.

Kathy wondered if she'd ever travel again; if she'd get to visit her daughter in Colorado.

Everything seemed so very hopeless.

Fortunately, Kathy was never any good at feeling sorry for herself. What she was especially good at was researching and solving problems.

One morning, she wrote on her white board, in large, bold letters: "I AM GOING TO BEAT THIS MONSTER WITHIN ME!"

Armed with a library card and access to the Internet, she started doing research. Most of what she found, primarily in medical reports and neurology journals, reinforced the hopelessness of her situation. Everyone had the same story; we have this great idea and if it works we'll be testing it with mice in a few years and then, assuming we get the funding, we'll move on to trials with humans and if that proves to be effective it may be available to the public in 10 or 15 years.

The life expectancy for a person with ALS is three to five years.

Kathy broadened her net and started looking in other

places. Near the end of the summer of 2006, she came across information that changed our lives: she discovered that there were, in fact, people who believed and had demonstrated that the progression of ALS could be halted and even reversed. These folks, outside of the established medical system, believed that the pharmaceutically-trained physicians, with their emphasis on drugs, were not only on the wrong track but may even be doing more harm.

The turf-protecting medical experts, on the other hand, seemed to consider anyone who advocated for healing without drugs to be a quack.

But the medical establishment didn't have a solution, only press releases about possible cures that loomed somewhere in a future that Kathy was not expected to see.

She kept reading and learning. Most of the alternative health care professionals agreed on one essential point: The key to healing neuromuscular disease was to rid the body of environmental poisons that had accumulated over the years; poisons from such things as pesticides, contaminated food, pharmaceutical drugs and, especially, mercury from dental fillings. All of these products contained neurotoxins—poisons that damage or destroy nerve cells.

It made sense. ALS is all about damaged nerve cells. Get rid of the reason the cells are being impaired and you've got a shot at recovery.

Since the medical establishment had nothing to offer us, we decided it was a waste of our time, energy and emotions to continue seeing them. We politely told them to take a flying leap.

Kathy stopped taking the medications that had been prescribed. I started buying only organic and locally grown foods. Together, we went through our home and tossed out all of the potentially toxic cleaning, personal hygiene and health care products.

She felt better almost instantly. Within days of stopping the drugs that had nearly paralyzed her face, she regained her lovely smile.

Hope.

Within a couple of weeks, we once again were going for long walks. By midwinter we were walking three and four miles at a time with no difficulty.

Kathy continued her research. One of the items strongly recommended was to have the amalgam fillings in her teeth removed. Amalgam fillings, often called silver fillings, are 52 percent mercury. Mercury is bad for you. We all know that. Mercury is banned from most products because it can do nasty things to your nervous system.

We asked our usual dentist to remove Kathy's fillings. He assured us that they were safe, no need to remove them.

Common sense seemed to indicate otherwise. Besides, even though Kathy had slowed the progression of her disease, she was still teetering on the brink of destruction. We'd rather err of the side of doing too much to help her than too little.

We began searching for a dentist who would remove the mercury fillings from Kathy's teeth. That was no easy task, especially since she couldn't swallow and the dental work would need to be done under general anesthesia.

During the next nine months, while we searched unsuccessfully for someone to safely remove the mercury from her mouth, she continued losing her strength, especially in her arms.

What she didn't lose was her determination to beat "this moldy old disease," as she'd begun calling it.

Eventually, in June 2007, we connected with the man who began the present-day campaign to ban mercury/amalgam fillings. He helped us arrange to get Kathy's fillings removed, and also worked very closely with us on monitoring and improving her blood chemistries. This was done through an even-more-restrictive diet, supplemented with minerals and vitamins. The goal was to remove the toxins that were in her system, while improving her body chemistry to the levels of someone who was in perfect health. In other words, give her body a chance to heal itself.

It began to work.

By October of 2007, Kathy was able to swallow small amounts of water. She hadn't swallowed anything since August of 2006. A short time later she began to sense small movements and tingling in her tongue. She hadn't moved her tongue in about a year and a half.

She was also beginning to regain some of the strength in her arms. Not much, but even small improvements let us know that she was finally heading in the right direction.

To say that Kathy was thrilled would be an understatement. It had taken a lot of searching and a lot of work, but it was beginning to pay off.

Unfortunately, Kathy's story doesn't have a happy ending.

In late October of 2007 she lost her balance while getting something out of the refrigerator and fell backward, hitting her head and wrenching her shoulder. She hadn't been sleeping very well for a long time, but after the fall—because of the pain in her shoulder and her inability to get comfortable—she could barely sleep at all.

That went on for three weeks. As she grew more and more tired, she also became more and more restless, to the point where she couldn't even get in a short nap.

Three weeks after the fall, Kathy died of exhaustion. During the last few days of her life she managed to get, maybe, three or four hours of sleep total, including nighttime and naps. None of it was restful.

Her last night, she was in and out of bed at least 20 times. Since she had very little use of her arms and limited leg strength, getting in and out of bed took a tremendous amount of her energy. She had the will to go on, but not the strength.

So, so sad.

Kathy knew that she was heading in the right direction. Her body was beginning to show improvements that the "experts" said were impossible. She had begun lifting light weights again and doing low-impact exercises to strengthen her legs and arms. She was enthralled at the feeling of cold water once again going down her throat.

Kathy was only 57. I will miss her dearly.

I've organized this book around the last week of Kathy's life. Throughout, I've provided flashbacks to help you better understand the entire journey that we took in search of healing from her disease.

My wish is that her story will help you recognize the fact that there is hope for folks with neuromuscular disease. If one life can be saved because of the things that Kathy learned and experienced, then maybe her journey will not have been in vain.

—*David Tank*

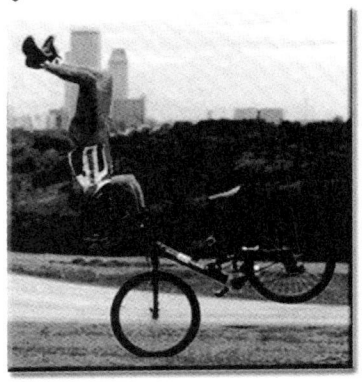

Life should **NOT** be a journey to the grave with the intention of arriving safely in an attractive and well preserved body, but rather to skid in sideways, champagne in one hand, strawberries in the other, body thoroughly used up, totally worn out and screaming WOO HOO! WHAT A RIDE!

Kathy created this mini-poster in 2004, shortly before her illness began, and from then on had it displayed prominently at each of her desks.

Original source of the quote and photo unknown.

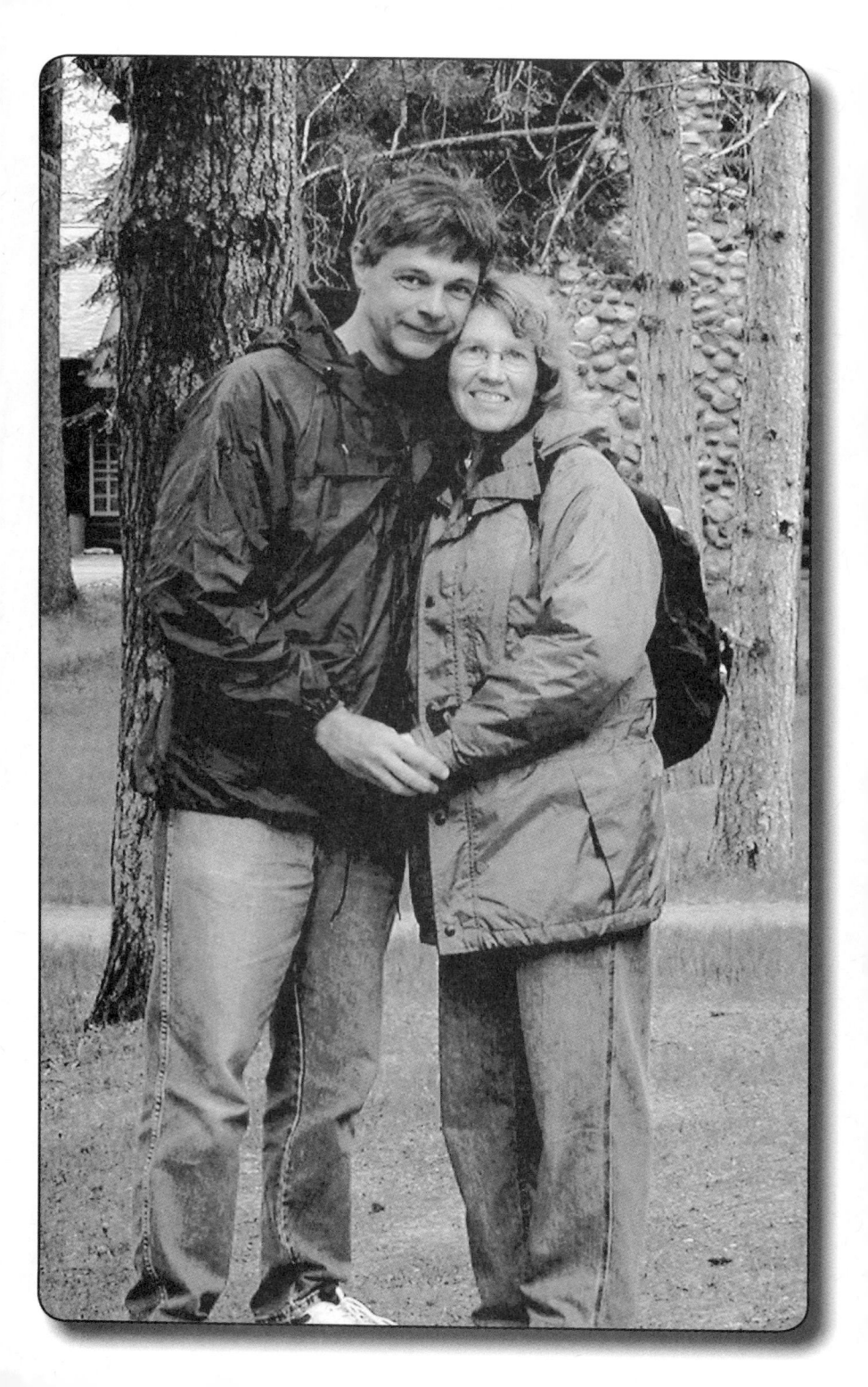

CHAPTER ONE
Tuesday, Nov. 6, 2007

"Hello Honey, I'm home."

I usually made that clichéd announcement when I walked in the back door after work. Very Ward Cleaverish. Sappy. Fun.

The day had gone okay for Kathy. I was at home with her through lunch. Keith, her youngest son, a senior at the local university, came over to spend the afternoon while I was at work at a different university, 20 miles away. Ann, our neighbor and Kathy's close friend, helped her with supper and stayed until I got back from the university at about 7:45.

Ever since her fall in the kitchen two weeks earlier, Kathy hated being home alone. We'd been figuring out ways to have people stay with her or stop in while I was at work.

Ann reported that the evening had gone well. She and Kathy had been talking about the healing power of humor. Ann said that she planned to pick up some funny movies at the library and bring them along on one of her next visits.

For the past two months, on Tuesday evenings when I had to work late, Ann stopped over to help Kathy with supper. It worked best if someone was at home to help her with her feeding tube.

On Monday nights, I would cook up an extra meal, liquefy

9

it in the blender, and store it in the refrigerator in a peanut butter jar. Then on Tuesday, when I was gone, Kathy would get the jar out of the refrigerator about 30 minutes before suppertime and set it in the sink in a bowl of hot water so that it would be warm by the time Ann arrived.

At first I put the liquefied meal in a glass canning jar, Kathy's preference for health reasons. But the weight of the glass was getting to be more than she could easily lift, so we switched to plastic. Besides being lighter, a plastic jar wouldn't break if she dropped it, which had happened once with glass.

Two weeks earlier, on Oct. 23, 2007, at about 4:30 p.m., as Kathy reached into the refrigerator to take out the jar of food, she lost her balance and tipped straight over backwards, grazing her head on the cupboard behind her and wrenching her neck. Her arms were too weak and too slow to break her fall. They also weren't strong enough to help her get up.

No one was home to help. She figured that if she could get to the stairway, on the other side of the dining room, she could use it to help raise herself.

Traversing the 25 feet across the dining room to the stairs was no easy task for her. Her arms were useless when it came to propelling herself across the coarse, Berber carpet, so she scooted her way across the room, using only her hips and legs. Eventually she made it to the bottom of the stairs, but she could not get herself up.

When Ann came in the back door 20 minutes later, she found the refrigerator door wide open, and on the far end of the dining room lay Kathy. She was exhausted. She had rug burns on her thighs. She'd wet herself.

Ann helped her up and steadied her as she walked to the bathroom and, after supper, to the couch.

At 6:13, using the laptop that sat on the small, portable table in front of the couch, Kathy sent me the following e-mail:

> i had a badday.fell and couldn' t ge tup orto aphn e .ann
> wilb here w heb u ge t hom e. k

One of our main methods of talking to each other was by e-mail. For years, when we were both at work, we'd e-mail each other several times a day, often just to flirt. After she lost her ability to speak, about a year and a half earlier, her computer and an array of whiteboards became her voice. Since we'd been sending e-mails to each other for years, that was a comfortable way of talking.

Often our messages crossed in cyberspace: We'd both hit SEND at the same time, without any idea that we were simultaneously at our computers. One of those times, she replied:

> don'tja just luv it when that happens!

I did.

Kathy had been the typing champion when she was in high school and people still marveled at her speed and accuracy. That skill had come in very handy when she lost her ability to speak.

As the disease progressed, it took its toll on her ability to move her fingers and her typing had begun to suffer. She was slowing down, to be sure. Sometimes she'd use text-messaging shortcuts to cut down on the number of key-strokes. But until her fall, she was still in control of the keyboard.

As I read her message the night that she fell, the quality of her typing, as well as her message, scared me.

> i had a badday.fell and couldn' t ge tup orto aphn e .ann
> wilb here w heb u ge t hom e. k

I had to read it a couple times to be sure what it said: "I had a bad day. Fell and couldn't get up or to a phone. Ann will be here when you get home. k."

Kathy and Ann were both pretty shaken when I arrived. Supper had gone okay, but Kathy was obviously in pain, both physically and emotionally. Lying on the floor, unable to get up or call for help, had scared her. What if it happened again? What if no one found her?

Even if she had been able to reach the phone, Kathy wondered how she would have told someone what happened, since she was unable to speak.

Before bed that night, I massaged Kathy's shoulders to help with the pain and stiffness that had already set in. Then we put an ice pack on the huge knot that had formed on her left shoulder.

When I washed her hair before bed, I discovered a large and tender bump on the top of her head. She was convinced that she'd only hit the floor when she fell, but from the placement of the bump on her skull and the distance between the refrigerator and the counter behind her, it was obvious that she'd also hit the cupboard door on the way down.

She used her white board and described the pain when she tried to lift her head as "a sharp stick poking into my neck, being twisted around." Her head hung down like the spent bloom of a week-old daisy.

Nearly three years earlier, in December 2004, Kathy first noticed something wrong with her tongue, but no one could tell her what caused it or what to do. Eighteen months later, when she was finally diagnosed with ALS, her tongue barely moved. It just sat uselessly on the floor of her mouth. By then, she also had great difficulty speaking and swallowing.

Kathy hadn't slept well in at least two years, not since the middle of 2005. At first it was because of medication that made her mouth so dry that she needed to wake up during the night to swab her lips and tongue with the little lollipop of a sponge strategically placed on the windowsill next to her bed. It wasn't unusual for her to wake up five or six times a night.

As her disease progressed, things changed and she was more likely to wake up during the night because she was choking on her saliva. In the daytime, the saliva often drooled uncontrollably from her mouth, making it uncomfortable for her to be out in public. She constantly had a cloth in her hand so that she could wipe her mouth and chin as needed.

At night, the saliva was often very thick and phlegmy. Since she couldn't swallow it and she didn't have the ability to spit it out, she'd have to keep going into the bathroom where she would literally pull the gunk out of her throat using a tongue brush. It wasn't unusual for the process to take 10 or 15 minutes. Several times it took more than an hour. She described it as "saliva hell."

Eventually, after a choking episode that lasted almost three hours and caused us to seriously consider calling 911, I ordered a portable vacuum pump, designed specifically for things like this. It didn't work.

So I rigged up a vacuum system of my own design, using a mini ShopVac and vinyl tubing. After we tested it out, I built it into the bathroom wall next to the sink, so it was always available.

That made the process a little easier and safer, but not any more pleasant. If the phlegm was stuck far down her throat, Kathy would still need to reach in with the tongue scraper and pull the glob up higher, before she could suck it out with the vacuum. What came out often resembled thick, stringy egg white. Sometimes the throat scraper would cause her to gag and vomit.

That went on for months, until in the fall of 2007 she discovered a simple change in the amount of salt and potassium in her diet that released her from saliva hell. Once the saliva problem was under control, she began to sleep a little better. She'd still get up to use the bathroom about every hour and a half to two hours and still needed to do a small amount of suctioning, but she felt that she had made it through the worst.

Healing had begun.

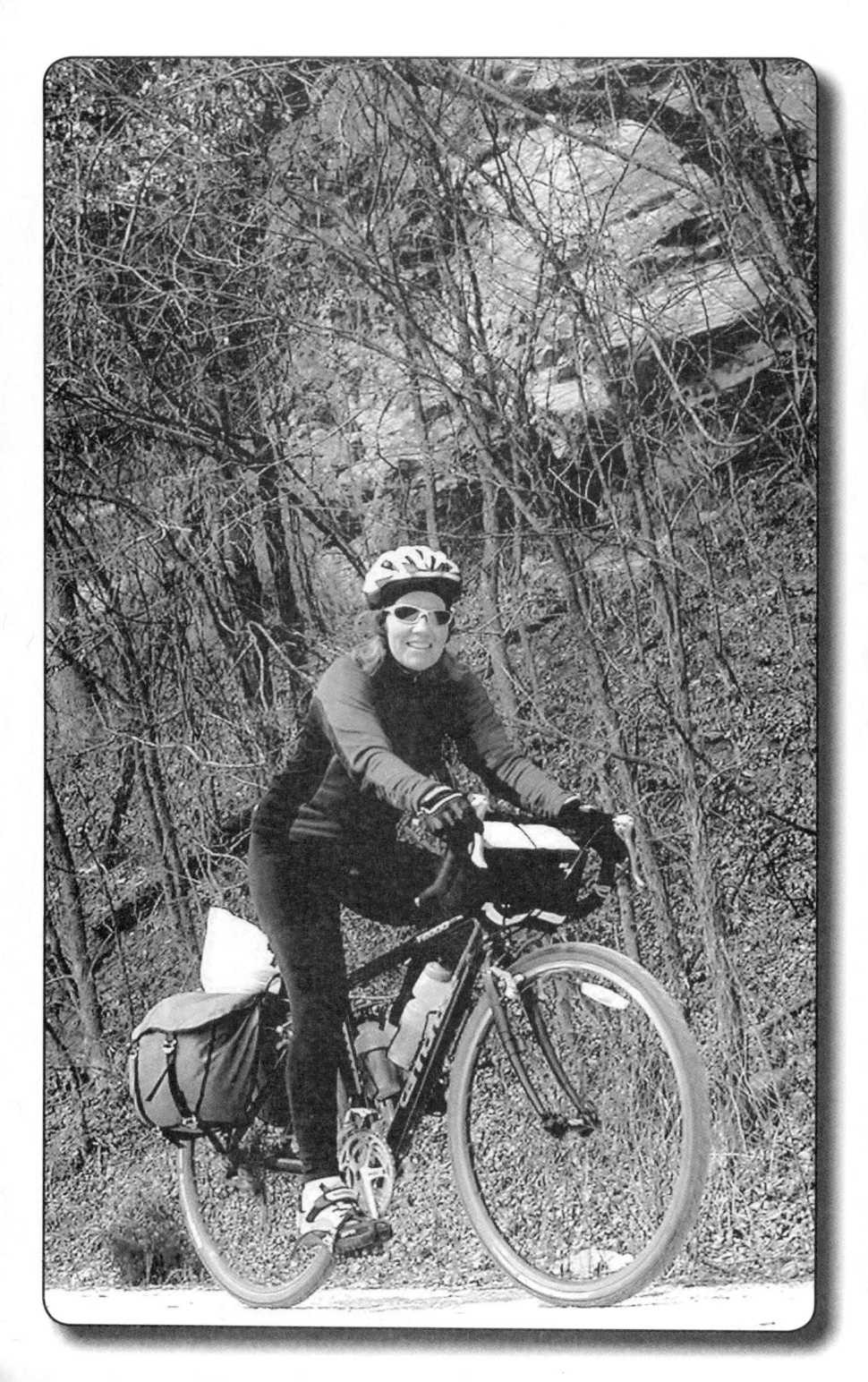

CHAPTER TWO
A Picture of Health

I've never known anyone who took better care of herself than Kathy. She rode her bicycle to work. She lifted weights. She cross-country skied and played racquetball.

Her diet consisted of fresh fruits and vegetables, whole-wheat bread and low-fat meats. Fast-food was almost never eaten. Her favorite beverages were water, jasmine tea and skim milk.

Kathy never smoked and actively avoided places with second-hand smoke. Her alcohol consumption consisted of locally produced wine, maybe once a week with a meal, and an occasional beer on a hot summer day.

For Kathy, getting wild and crazy meant having a Dr Pepper and a small bag of M&M's. She did everything she could to stay in good health and top physical condition.

I often wondered if the reason Kathy worked so hard to maintain her health was so she didn't end up like her mother, in a wheelchair for 30 years from rheumatoid arthritis. I remember Kathy once saying, after we'd hiked to a hard-to-reach summit with an unbeatable view, "I wish that my mother would have been able to experience a view like this." Actually, she'd said that a number of times. She always felt that her mom got robbed by not being able to physically enjoy the things that she loved.

Few of the activities that Kathy participated in were competitive. That's probably good because when Kathy did compete, she was determined to win. Giving up or quitting were not in her nature.

One of her favorite magazines was "Silent Sports," which featured articles about such things as hiking, biking and cross-country skiing, the sorts of sports that let you quietly enjoy the outdoors and the things that are in it.

One of our favorite activities together was canoeing. Living in Wisconsin, we had many incredible rivers to choose from, all within a few hours of our home, and we paddled many of them. Kathy wasn't a fan of canoeing on lakes. She liked to be close to the bank so she could enjoy a water-level view of the plants and animals that lived there.

Kathy's favorite river was the Namekagon, a narrow, wild and scenic river that always had good water levels. We paddled it every year, sometimes a couple of times so we could enjoy watching it change with the seasons.

Another set of rivers that we loved were what we called the "P" rivers; the Peshtigo, Popple, Pine and Pike. They were a bit more challenging and included some pretty good rapids. Not far away were the Prairie and the Pelican.

We tried them all, but our favorite was the Peshtigo. We maneuvered our way through its rocky, twisting course three or four times. The Peshtigo was the first river to ever get the best of us. We capsized at a rapids so challenging that just downstream we found someone else's bent and twisted canoe and, just beyond that, a kayak wedged under a fallen tree. We were proud that we'd done better than their crews. Aside from some bruises to our bodies and spirits, the only thing we lost were a water bottle and Kathy's favorite cap.

When you canoe on a river, one problem is shuttling from the end of the trip back to the beginning, where you left your car. Many people canoe with friends or in groups so that one vehicle can be parked at the take-out spot, providing a way back to the starting point.

Occasionally we'd do that. But our preference was to canoe alone so we'd have a better chance of seeing the undisturbed wildlife. Besides, we enjoyed the company of each other more than being part of a group.

Rather than take two cars, we would take along our bikes. We'd drop off the canoe at the starting point, then drive to the take-out location. We'd leave the vehicle there, then bicycle back to our canoe. It worked great and made for an enjoyable day. A typical trip might be 12 miles of canoeing and eight miles of biking.

For Kathy, eight miles of biking was like paddling with the wind at your back. When she was in her 20s, she toured the United States and Canada by bike. In 1976 she was a tour leader for one of the cross-country Bike Centennial tours, riding more than 3,000 miles. Thirty years later, she still had her biking legs.

Kathy's love of the outdoors was also evident in other areas. She was a Master Gardener, Master Composter and, for the five years before her illness, had her own gardening business called The Garden Tender. Her favorite customers were the older folks; those who had tended their own gardens for many years, but were now finding it difficult to manage without help. Sometimes she'd work alongside them, doing the more difficult tasks. Other times she'd take on the whole project, and often chat with them while she worked. Many of these folks thought of her more as a friend than as a hired gardener.

Her own gardens in our yard were spectacular. When we bought our house in 1992, the landscaping included only one tiny rock garden. Fifteen years later the yard was totally transformed, with thousands of flowers in a dozen unique settings.

Working together on her gardens helped establish the way that we would work together later to challenge her illness. Kathy was generally the idea person. She was constantly learning new things about gardening and enjoyed reading, attending workshops and swapping ideas with friends.

Once she had an idea of what she wanted, she'd try to convey her vision to me. That wasn't always easy, because my gardening experience pretty much consisted of marigolds in a foot-wide bed along the side of the house. Fortunately, she was a good and patient teacher. Once we decided what we were going to do, my primary role was to till up the new beds and build any needed structures, such as arbors or fences.

One thing that we were especially good at was building on each other's ideas. A perfect example was the time she said that she'd like a higher vantage point from which to look into our little pond. I started with an idea for a small platform. She said, "Great. What if we tried a raised walkway." I countered, "How about if we expand the walkway to include a raised area for a little table" After a couple of months and many "what-if-we-tried" discussions, our humble little platform evolved into a 14-by-14-foot tree house, complete with a bed, a dining area, easy chairs and its own front deck overlooking the pond.

Given free reign, we could produce amazing results and have a lot of fun doing it. We often amazed ourselves at just how far we were willing to take a project before we were satisfied. "Good enough" was a phrase that we'd consciously banned from our vocabularies early in our marriage.

In the colder months, when Kathy couldn't get outside as often, she quilted. Of course, she didn't just make simple quilts to put on a bed. She custom-designed artistic quilts, with such perfect hand-stitching that it was impossible to see the difference in size from one stitch to the next. She prided herself on her perfection, without ever bragging about it.

Kathy was already an accomplished quilter when we met, and she had exhibited her work in juried quilt shows. I was impressed with what she'd done. One day she showed me a wall quilt that she'd started but had given up on. I thought it looked a bit too proper and asked if she could make the quilt look more three-dimensional and more fun. She took on the challenge, but only if I was willing to help her redesign it.

My contributions to that quilting project were mostly in the form of "what-if-you-tried" statements. Even so, and in spite of the fact that I seweth not one stitch, she included my name on the signature block that she attached to the back of the quilt. A few months later she entered it in a quilt show and won first prize in a category created just for "our" quilt—most whimsical.

Without realizing it, a team had been born.

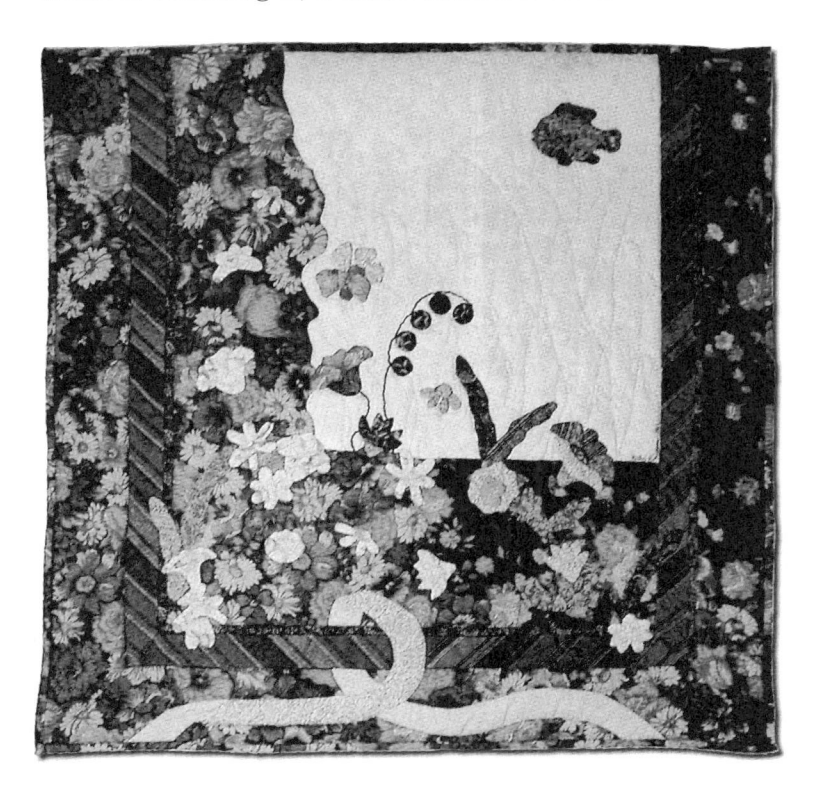

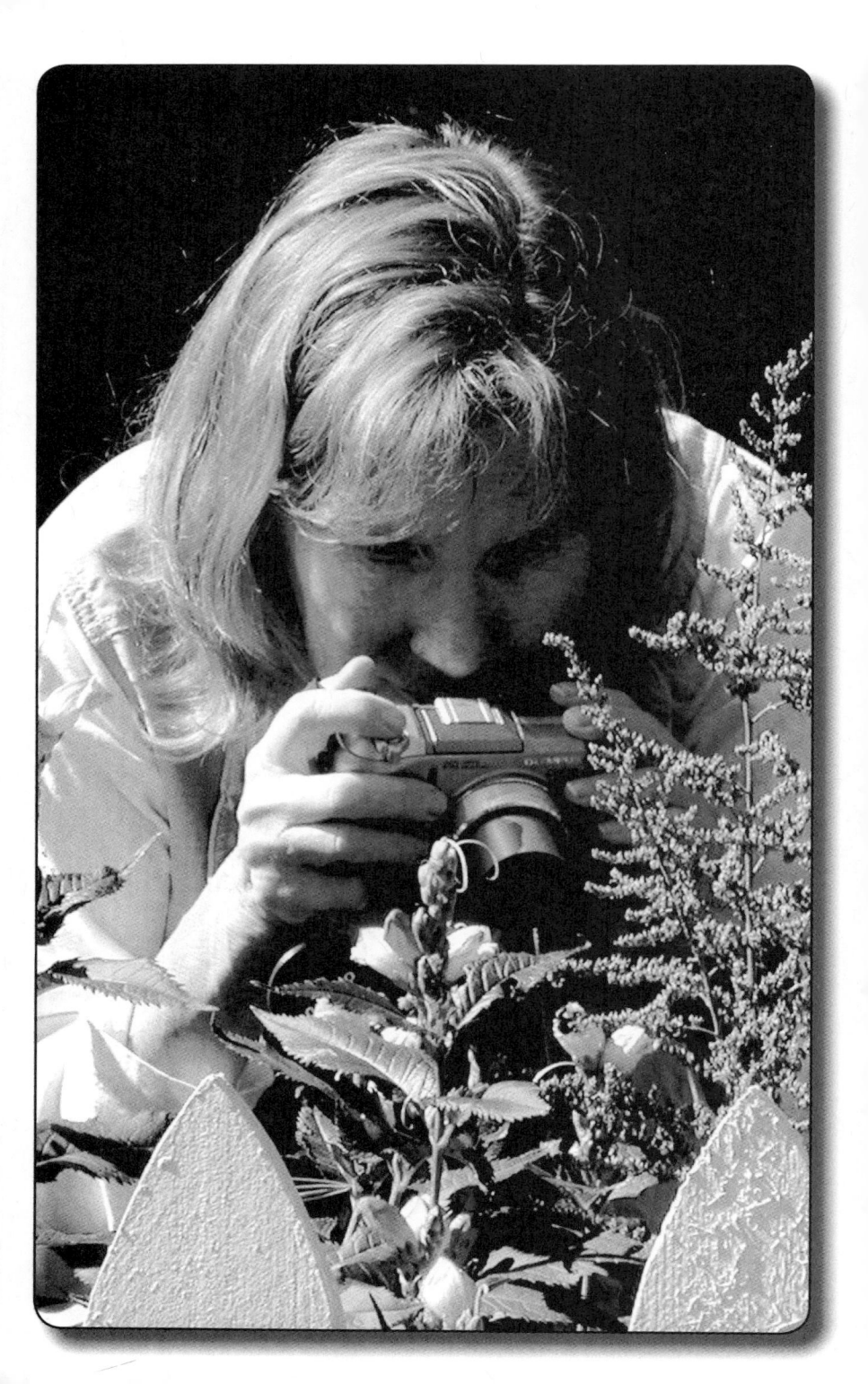

CHAPTER THREE
"A Cold Drink of Water is Heavenly"

Beginning in early September of 2007, about seven weeks before her fall in the kitchen, Kathy began to recover her ability to swallow, something we'd been told by the experts was impossible. After not swallowing anything in many months she was exhilarated. She wrote to me and many of her friends, "A cold drink of water is HEAVENLY."

She had worked her way up to it slowly. Trying to drink from a glass or a cup was difficult for several reasons. For one thing, a cup filled with water was too heavy for her to lift to her lips. When she did get the cup to her mouth, the water usually poured out too fast and she'd quickly have to tip the cup back up. But most importantly, when she tipped her head back to drink, her wind pipe would be opened and the water would splash into her trachea causing her to choke.

Nonetheless, by the end of summer she was convinced that she would be able to drink again. I'm not sure what it was, but something inside of her seemed to be saying, *now is the time for you to start swallowing.*

She sent me out to Shopko to buy some training cups for toddlers. I came home with a couple different levels. Each restricted the amount of water that flowed from them to a different degree. The toddler cups were also smaller, lighter and designed to be easily held. They were an improvement, but she still needed to tip her head back, opening up her wind pipe. Try as she might, she didn't manage to get a single drop down her throat.

She tried a straw. That didn't work at all because she couldn't close her lips around it tight enough to create any suction. Instead, she ended up crushing the straw with her teeth. So she sent me back to the baby section at Shopko to find a stronger straw.

This time I came home with a green, spill-proof glass that had a bright-blue, heavy-duty, removable straw sticking out of the top. Kathy gave that a try. She didn't crush it with her teeth, but she still wasn't able to get enough suction to pull any liquid up into her mouth.

Then she came up with the idea of using a siphon. It would be like a straw, but she would not need to suck on it to get the liquid into her mouth. She also wouldn't need to tip her head back.

As so often was the case, she came up with the idea and then turned it over to me to figure out how to implement. Fortunately, we seldom threw anything away.

When Kathy first had her feeding tube put in, we poured the cans of formula into special bags, called gravity bags. The bags were designed to hang from a pole, just like the bags for a blood transfusion, and each bag had attached a length of tubing with a shut-off valve. We'd stopped using the bags shortly after we got them, when we switched over to liquefying real food in the blender. The unused bags were still in a box in the basement.

I cut a small length of tubing from one of the unused gravity bags and brought it upstairs. Kathy sat down at the kitchen counter with a towel on her lap and a smile on her face. She just knew that this was going to work.

I stood next to Kathy and inserted one end of the tube into a large mug filled with water and held it higher than her head. Then I gently sucked on the siphon to get the action started and handed the end of the tube to her.

She directed the small stream into her mouth without

tipping her head back. Most of it ended up on her shirt, on the counter and on the floor, but she ended up swallowing a few drops without choking. Only a few drops. But when you haven't swallowed anything in months, a few drops is pretty exciting.

After that, she wanted to practice over and over. But, to be very honest, I didn't have the extra time each day to stand there holding the cup in the air. I tried rigging it up on a little stand, but that didn't work very well.

Eventually, it occurred to me that instead of cutting the tubing off of the gravity bag to use for a siphon, why not use the whole thing as a water delivery system.

I filled one of the bags with distilled water and hung it above the bathroom sink, so that Kathy could get a drink whenever she wanted. She could use the little slider valve at the end of the hose to start and stop the flow. My job was to keep the bag filled with water.

It was an overnight success. And I mean that quite literally. When she'd get up in the night to use the toilet, she'd also enjoy a little water.

At first, most of the water was still running back out of her mouth, down her arms and chin and into the sink or onto the floor. But each day her swallowing muscles got stronger.

I would often help hold the tube up for her when her arms got tired, and I could watch the muscles in her throat expand and contract as she swallowed. Absolutely thrilling. Even though much of the water was running down her neck and chin, it was obvious that more water was going into her mouth than was running back out.

Within a couple of weeks I was having a hard time staying ahead of her on keeping the bag filled. That was especially frustrating for her when I wasn't there to refill it, so I added a second hook and hung up a second bag. That way she had at least two bags of water available. The more that she practiced her drinking, the faster the bags were emptied.

As exciting as it was, this bit of progress was becoming

frustrating for both of us: for her because the bags so often went dry, and for me because it seemed that refilling them had become a never-ending task.

Finally I tapped into the water line, added a small valve at the front of the sink and attached a piece of tubing that would deliver the water slowly at low pressure. Besides the obvious advantage of a never-ending supply, she also discovered that by letting it run for awhile she could drink the water ice cold. The water in the bags had been room temperature.

From then on, she got a drink nearly every time she went into the bathroom. Sometimes she'd stay in there 10 or 15 minutes enjoying the feel of the water going down her throat.

The cold water did odd things to her saliva, causing it to get thicker. But that was easily solved with the suction tube, which stuck out of the wall only a few inches above the water tube. In a way that I never could have appreciated before, life was good. Things were moving forward.

Swallowing wasn't the only progress that Kathy was making. The week before her fall in the kitchen, she made another, even more exciting advancement.

When Kathy got up to use the toilet at night—which was more often since she was getting a drink each time she was there—her first stop on returning to the bedroom would be to stand next to my side of the bed so that I could reach out and help pull up her pajamas. She'd do this as quietly as possible so that she wouldn't wake me any more than necessary. She knew that once I was wide awake I had a hard time getting back to sleep. She also knew, from experience, that if I was awakened quickly I could be pretty grumpy.

But that mid-October night, as I she stood next to my side of the bed, she flipped on the light on my night stand as bright as it would go, leaned over and stared into my eyes like a crazy woman.

"What the heck are you... ?"

Before I could finish, she bent down and gave me the happiest, sloppiest kiss I've ever had. Then she grabbed her white board and wrote: "MY TONGUE MOVED!"

Her tongue hadn't moved in more than a year. Not even a little. Believe me, I wasn't the slightest bit grumpy that she woke me up so suddenly. First her swallowing, now her tongue. Everything that we'd been working so hard at to help her body heal itself was beginning to pay off.

The next day she began feeling a tingling in her tongue, a sensation she described as being much the same as the feeling that you get after your foot falls asleep. The nerves in her tongue were waking up, once again beginning to function.

We'd been told that was impossible, too.

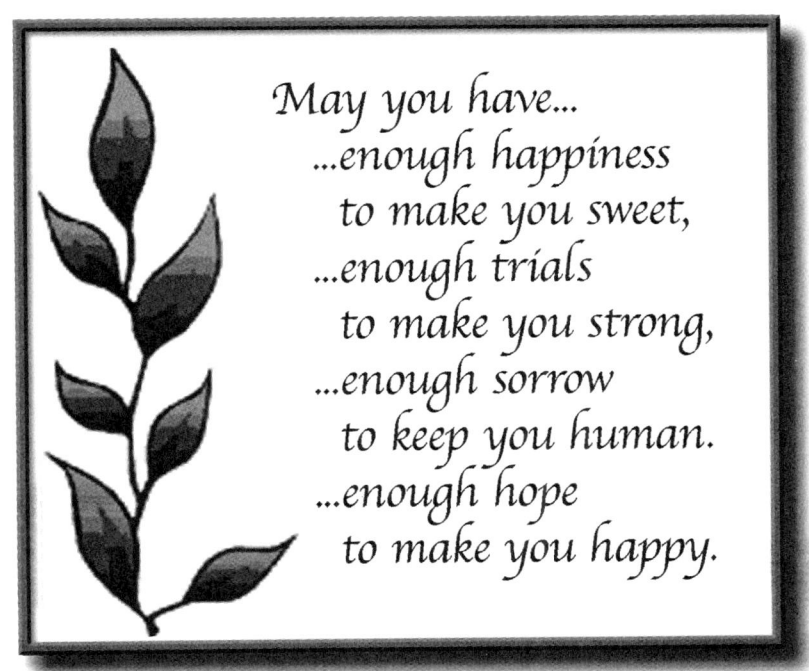

May you have...
...enough happiness
to make you sweet,
...enough trials
to make you strong,
...enough sorrow
to keep you human.
...enough hope
to make you happy.

From Kathy's personal home page. Original author unknown.

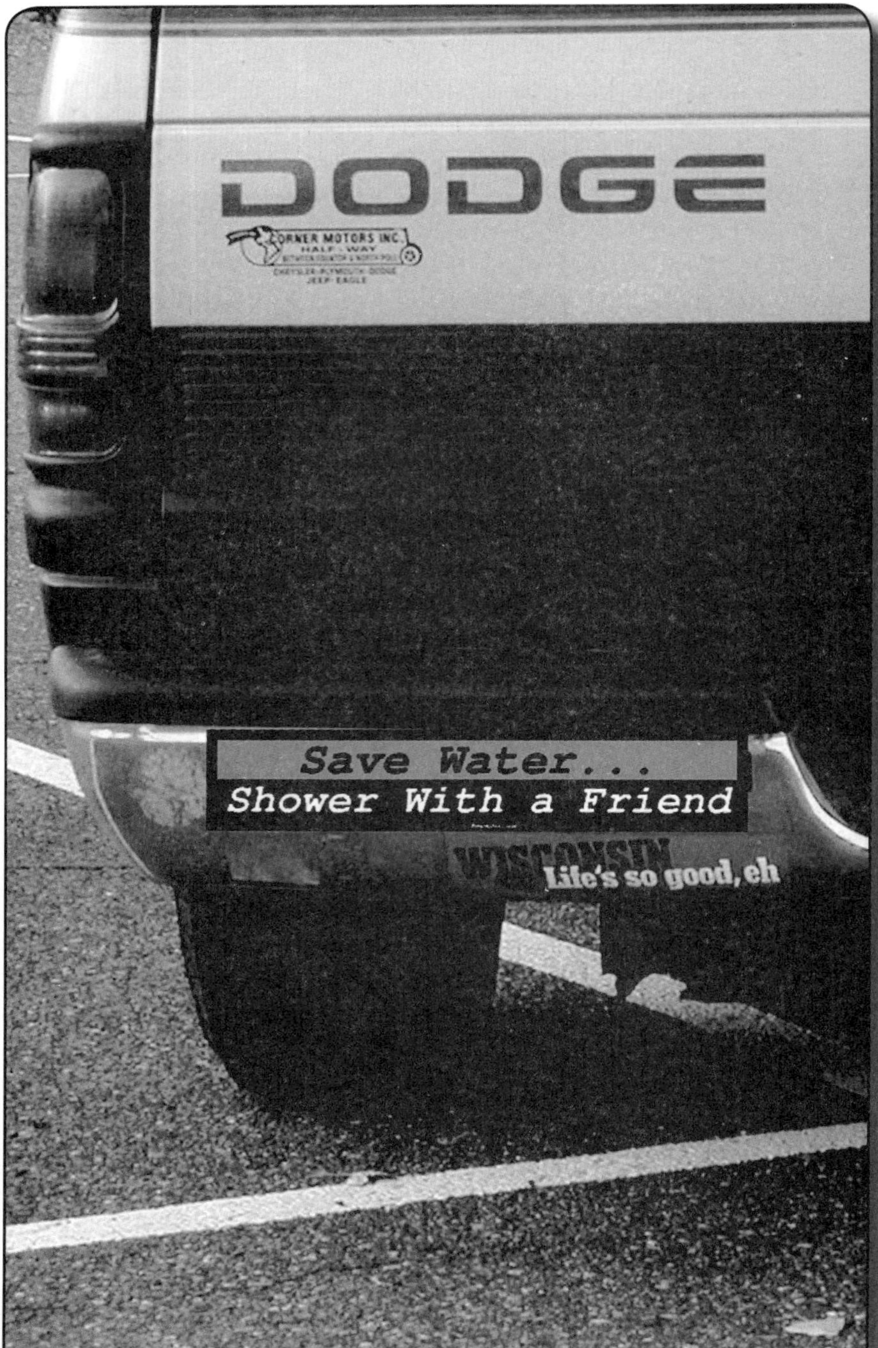
DODGE
Save Water...
Shower With a Friend
Life's so good, eh

CHAPTER FOUR
Save Water, Shower With a Friend

When I got home from school on Tuesday, Nov. 6, 2007, Kathy seemed especially restless. Ann said that she'd been that way all evening. To help her relax, she'd been massaging Kathy's neck.

My being home seemed to have a calming effect on Kathy. She had gotten to the point in the last week or so where she didn't want me out of her sight any more than absolutely necessary.

"I've become a Klingon," she wrote, knowing that I was an old Star Trek fan. Even though we'd always enjoyed each other's company, clinging on was new for her.

At her request, several days earlier, I'd moved my computer into the dining room from my basement office so that I would be closer to her when I did my schoolwork.

That Tuesday evening, we sat on the couch and I rubbed her shoulders and feet as we watched the latest episode of "House," an offbeat show about an unconventional doctor who could find a cure for just about anything if he worked at it long enough. It was one of our favorite shows and we always watched it together. If I wasn't home when the program started, Kathy would tape it so that we could watch it later.

Together, we were a lot like an episode of "House." We were

not willing to give up on solving Kathy's medical dilemma until we had exhausted every possible avenue of helping her heal. Sometimes we had to try unconventional approaches. But we knew that by the end of the episode, with research and diligence, we could beat this monster within her. The recent improvements in her health intensified our hope that her efforts would eventually pay off.

After Dr. House solved his latest patient's unsolvable illness, it was time for our nightly shower. We'd been showering together since May. Care giving does have its benefits.

In about March of 2007, I'd begun helping Kathy wash her hair because it was getting difficult for her to reach the top of her head. By May we'd decided that the most efficient way to handle this was to simply shower together.

The nightly shower quickly became a ritual. She'd head off to her bathroom alone to take care of the preliminaries and start warming up the water in the shower. The single, round shower knob had become difficult to grip, making it hard for her to adjust the temperature and flow, so I added an extension lever. It didn't look great, but it made it possible for her to get the shower started without my help.

After she was in the shower, I'd step into the bathroom, politely knock on the glass shower door, then join her. Fitting two people into Kathy's tiny shower was a pleasant challenge. Her shower was so small that when I needed to replace the shower door, I ended up having to buy the store's undersized sample.

Since there wasn't a lot of room to maneuver, showering had to be carefully choreographed. If I reached for the shampoo the wrong way, she'd end up with an elbow to her nose. If she turned around too quickly, I'd get a boob in the belly. The fact that we enjoyed being close was about the only thing that made it work. Sometimes it was even fun.

The weight of a wet washcloth was more than Kathy could lift above her shoulders, so the first thing I'd do was help her wash her face. I was worried that I'd get soap in her eyes, and she was concerned that if I did get soap in her eyes she wouldn't have an easy way to let me know or to rinse it out.

So the first part of our little dance went like this: She would face the wall and I would stand behind her. As I soaped up the washcloth, she would bend her arms at the elbows, put her hands together and slowly raise them, using the shower wall as a sort of slide. I'd then place the washcloth over her hands, put my hands under her elbows, and raise her arms until her hands reached her face.

By simply helping to hold her arms up, she was able to wash her face herself. When she was finished, she'd flip the washcloth onto her shoulder so I'd know that she was done. While I was getting the washcloth ready for the next sequence of the dance, she'd slide her arms back down the wall and turn her head toward the shower to rinse off her face. It worked pretty well. I only recall getting soap in her eyes once, and she handled it without complaint.

Once she started swallowing again, she added another move to this little section of the dance. She opened her lips as she rinsed her face and let the water run into her mouth, swallowing a few drops. There was very little that pleased her more than feeling the drops of water run down her throat and she took advantage of any opportunity that she could.

While she was thus distracted, I'd move on to the rest of her body. The trickiest part was washing around her feeding tube. Until about the time that she fell in the kitchen, she preferred doing that herself.

The tube wasn't stitched in—it stayed in place pretty much by the strength of her stomach and abdominal muscles. A small amount of waxy matter, somewhat like ear wax, would leak out around the tube where it entered her body and this needed to be cleaned off every night.

She'd usually use the tip of her finger to do this in the shower, under the running water. Of course getting the sticky gunk off of her finger was the next problem. For some unknown reason she'd taken to wiping it onto my hairy thigh, and let me worry about what to do with it from there. At first, I thought it was because my leg was the closest and handiest thing for her to use. But later I decided that she did it just for the fun of annoying me.

The last sequence was shampooing her hair. I think that we both enjoyed that part of the dance. I especially enjoyed running the comb through her hair after I'd applied the conditioner.

Kathy had gorgeous, blond hair and always took exceptionally good care of it. She enjoyed enhancing its natural beauty with clips and barrettes. For the last few years she had been keeping it long.

As her arms became weaker, it became more and more difficult for her to comb out and style her hair herself. Ever resourceful, she discovered that if she kneeled on the bedroom floor in front of her dressing table, which had a mirror at the right height, and rested her elbows on the top of the table, she could maneuver the comb and brush satisfactorily. She'd been doing that for some time without me seeing her, so I was a little slow in realizing that she'd lost her ability to reach the top of her head.

About the same time that I started washing her hair, she decided to have it cut shorter so that it was easier to manage. For years she'd gone to the same hair stylist. But when she learned that chemical toxins may have helped cause her illness, she felt that it was no longer safe to go into her usual hair salon.

By searching through the phone book and making a few calls, we managed to find a sweet, older woman who had a small styling shop in the basement of her home. She was willing to schedule Kathy at times when no one else was there or had an appointment before her, so there would be no fumes from permanents or hair spray in the room.

Since Kathy couldn't speak, she took along pictures she'd cut from magazines to show the woman the way she would like her hair cut. With the use of her white board, they managed to carry on the usual hair salon chatter quite nicely.

After her fall in the kitchen, because she couldn't hold her head up, Kathy had a harder time combing her hair, even when on her knees in front of the mirror, so taking care of her tresses became almost exclusively my responsibility.

I was just awful at it.

Even though her hair was, by then, quite short, I could not figure out what she did to make it look so nice. A couple of times she had me hold her hand in mine as I combed her hair, and she tried to steer me in the right direction. That actually worked fairly well. A little flip here and a short stroke there and she looked pretty good.

But when I tried to do the same thing on my own it always came out looking pretty much like my hair, which was nothing to brag about. How she put up with my inept hair styling, without showing me the slightest bit of disgust, I'll never know. She just shook her head in a way that said, "That's my David. I love him anyway."

When we were finished showering, I would usually step out of the shower first and greet her with a towel as she stepped out behind me. I'd hold the towel open and she'd lean forward so that her face was in it and position her hands under it. I'd help her hold her hands in place and when she straightened up the towel went with her and she was able to dry her face.

I was in charge of drying her hair and the rest of her body. I learned early on that hair needed to be dried first or it would keep dripping onto the parts of her body that I'd already dried. Efficiency was everything.

After she was dry, there were several creams and ointments that I'd apply, all of them natural or organic. Each had a different purpose and location. The basic skin lotion was for her back and legs. Another, specially compounded by a women's health pharmacy with some sort of special hormone in it, was rubbed into the small of her back.

Then some slimy stuff, called Muscle Rescue Gel, went onto her arms and shoulders. And finally, a tiny amount of Burt's Bees diaper cream was gently applied just below where her feeding tube entered her belly.

She'd made herself some small, soft, flannel pads that fit around the base of the tube so that it wouldn't chafe against her skin. We'd originally purchased disposable pads specifically designed for this purpose, but it didn't take long before Kathy decided she could fashion something that was more comfortable, worked better and wasn't so wasteful.

The feeding tube, called a PEG tube, short for percutaneous endoscopic gastrostomy, was very flexible and hung out of her abdomen like an umbilical cord. To keep it out of the way, she or I simply tucked it into the waist band of her pants or underpants, whichever worked better.

At the end of the tube was an oddly shaped cap, where the tube could be connected to the syringe. The feel of the cap rubbing against her waist was annoying, so she also made a flannel cover for it—kind of like a little mitten without a thumb. It had the added benefit of keeping the tube from accidentally popping open. That had happened once shortly after she got the tube, spewing her stomach contents like a squirt gun as she ran from the bathroom to the kitchen for my help.

Next she weighed herself. We both kept track of her weight. She didn't have the same sense of hunger using the feeding tube, so the best way to know that she was getting the right amount of food was to keep an eye on the scale. She monitored it every evening after her shower to the tenth of a pound.

Before she got her PEG tube, her weight had gone down to about 104. For the past year she'd been maintaining it at about 113.6, just about perfect for her 5-foot-3-inch frame.

On that Tuesday night, two weeks after her fall, however, her weight was a little higher. She had started to retain fluid in her ankles and feet the past couple days. It wasn't a lot, but it was enough of a concern that we decided to cut back on the amount of salt in her diet.

For the first 10 months after she got her feeding tube, it took four meals a day to keep her weight at that optimal level. Shortly after we revised her diet, in June of 2007, we were able to cut back to three meals a day. That worked much better for both of us.

We had always enjoyed sharing our meals together, usually with a nicely set table and candles. We played a little game to see who could come up with the most creative way to lay out the place-settings. You'd be amazed at how many variations are possible once you break away from what's expected.

Even when we ate on the porch, which was anytime the weather was warm, or in the tree house, when we just felt like having fun, we'd set the table nicely and enjoy each other's company.

That didn't work so well when Kathy first got her tube. Initially she was using the prescribed, canned formula. For that, she'd need to sit in a chair for 45 minutes, tethered to the gravity bag, which slowly dripped the "food" into her system.

The bag needed to be hung higher than her head for it to work properly. A portable, aluminum pole with a chrome hook came with the program. Boring. And actually, not all that stable.

So we rigged up a couple of other hooks. One was on her office wall, above her desk, so she could work at her computer while she feasted. Another, fashioned from a wrought iron plant hanger, was placed in the garden next to Kathy's favorite Adirondack chair. We even rigged up a hook in my truck so that she could enjoy a delicious formula treat while we traveled. Yum.

I probably shouldn't make too much fun of the formula. It did quickly build up Kathy's weight when we had no other options. And the insurance company paid for it!

However, reading the ingredients on the can was like looking at the contents of my childhood chemistry set. The only things that sounded even remotely like food were fractionated coconut and palm kernel oil, canola oil, corn oil and salt.

As soon as her weight stabilized, we switched over to blending our own food. Everything Kathy ate from then on was organic and cooked from scratch. To eliminate the possibility of adding such potentially dangerous elements as aluminum and nickle into her system, we got rid of all of our metal cookware and replaced it with glass. Nothing was microwaved. Most of the vegetables were steamed fresh and most of the meat, usually turkey, was baked.

Kathy's meals and my meals were pretty much identical, except mine would go onto a plate and hers would go into the blender.

Instead of sitting at the table, we'd stand at the kitchen counter. Most of the time, especially during the first year after her tube was installed, Kathy handled the tube feeding on her own and it was easier for her to do that standing up. My job was to make the food, blend it, and pour it into a jar on the counter. She then took over, pulling the mixture into a large syringe and squeezing it out into her tube.

We usually watched the 5:30 national news during mealtime or, if I was slow in cooking, the 6 p.m. local news. It wasn't that hard for us to act as if things were back to normal, with one exception: We never did figure out any creative place-settings for the feeding tube.

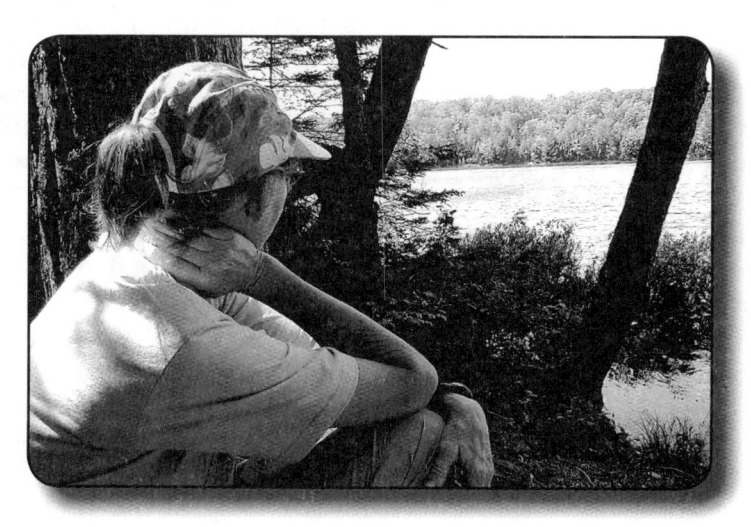

CHAPTER FIVE
Bedtime—Let the Torture Begin

"Ready for the torture to begin?" I asked. It was Tuesday, Nov. 6, 2007, about 10:15 p.m., two weeks to the day after Kathy had fallen in the kitchen. She nodded slightly. Slowly. Reluctantly.

Neither of us was ever ready for bed anymore. We simply knew that sooner or later it was something that we had to do. Bedtime no longer offered any rest. Nights had become something to endure, something to try to make it to the end of with minimal damage and frustration. Each morning we got up more tired than when we'd gone to bed the night before.

We used to watch the Channel 18 news every night at 10 and go to bed immediately after the weather. But in the past few weeks, we'd begun to leave the TV on and switch to Jay Leno; partly to stall, partly to get a bit of humor into our souls before the nighttime torture began.

Bedtime used to be a special time for us. For as long as we were married, we seldom went to bed alone unless I was working late in my basement office reading manuscripts. We'd usually turn off the TV, each head into our own bathroom, return to our bedroom at about the same time, and crawl into bed.

Once we turned off the lights, I'd say "Good night Kathy, I love you." Sometimes she responded with "me too you."

Other times she'd put her hand on my thigh or maybe touch my foot with her toe. Then we'd take each other's hand and fall asleep.

I was always a little jealous of how quickly she could nod off. She could close her eyes, somehow tell herself to go to sleep, and almost instantly be in slumber land. If she couldn't get to sleep within five minutes she was frustrated; she would roll over or maybe even get up to use the toilet again.

I, on the other hand, routinely lay in bed for 20 to 30 minutes, replaying everything I'd done that day and planning for what would greet me tomorrow.

We'd done that same bedtime ritual, or some slight variation of it, for years. It always started with me telling her I loved her. It always ended with us holding hands.

The day that I told my older brother that I was going to marry Kathy, he gave me some advice: "Never let a day go by without telling her that you love her. It'll let *her* know, and remind *you*." Good advice. Sometimes I told her twice.

Since the summer, we'd quietly reworked that ritual, adapting it as her illness progressed.

More recently, the first step of going to bed was for me to help Kathy get started in the bathroom. She would walk into her bathroom ahead of me. Then, a minute or so later I would show up knocking at the door.

I didn't "take her to the bathroom." She went in on her own and I stopped by to help—a subtle difference that was never discussed, but understood and appreciated by both of us. Early on in her disease she said to me, "I'm afraid that I'm going to lose all of my dignity." I did my best to keep that from happening.

Once we were inside the bathroom together, I gently slid her pajamas down over her hips, making sure not to catch the feeding tube. I slid them down just far enough so that she could hook her thumbs into their waistband and finish pulling them down herself after I left. Sometimes I helped her raise her thumbs a little higher, rather than pull down her pajama bottoms a bit lower.

The amount of help she needed with her pajamas was a good way for me to gauge the progression of her disease. Until the summer of 2007, I didn't need to help her pull down her pajamas at all. In September, I only needed to pull them down an inch or two. But the distance increased rapidly after her fall. It was getting more and more difficult for Kathy to raise her hands even as high as her lower hips.

Once she hooked her thumbs onto her pajama bottoms I would leave, gently pulling the bathroom door almost closed. A piece of duct tape over the latch, placed there by Kathy a couple of months earlier, assured that it could not be closed tightly. Turning the small doorknob had become difficult for her and she feared being trapped in the bathroom. I offered to replace the knob with a lever that would be easier to open. In fact, one day I came home with one from the hardware store. She made me take it back. She didn't want me to start making changes to the house to accommodate her. That would be admitting defeat. The duct tape would be fine, and it could easily be removed when it was no longer needed.

After I left the bathroom, it was time for me to step over to the kitchen to prepare a lovely syringe of LiverMate.

LiverMate is a concoction developed by Doc Huggins to, as its name implies, help the liver. As we'd been told on more than one occasion, the human body has two things going for it: its liver and its kidneys. If both are working efficiently, you've got a good shot at recovering. If not, you don't have much of a chance to heal.

So every night I prepared the LiverMate. It was a simple process if you could swallow: Pop one capsule into your mouth and wash it down with a drink of water.

For us, it was a bit more complicated: Open one capsule of LiverMate; pour the gray contents into a small, shot-glass sized container with about an ounce of distilled water; cap the container and shake well.

Then I waited until Kathy rang a small school bell. That bell had once called her from recess at Catholic school back in Comfrey, Minnesota. Now it sat on a stool in her bathroom.

The bell was her signal for me to come back for her. Lately, she waited a long time to ring the bell, and I'd find her in front of the sink, her pajamas somewhere between her knees and her thighs, head hanging down over the basin, spraying water into her mouth from the little hose.

We never could determine how much water she was actually swallowing. She said that she couldn't tell for sure. She knew that it had gone beyond the initial few drops, but other than that she didn't know. One thing that we were sure of was that since I rigged up the drinking tube, she needed to use the bathroom more often.

I wanted to figure out a way to measure her intake. It seemed to me that I should know so that I could appropriately adjust the amount of water I was providing through her feeding tube. The one idea that I came up with, using a small wash basin to try to catch the water that ran back out of her mouth, and then compare that to the amount of water that flowed from the tube alone during the same amount of time, didn't work.

She didn't really care. She was just thrilled that she was swallowing anything.

Once I coaxed Kathy away from the water, I helped her with her pajamas. Getting her pajamas *up* was more difficult for her than pushing them *down*. Her arms were weaker when it came to pulling. So I would pull them up for her.

Since we were heading to the kitchen for her LiverMate, there was no need to tuck her feeding tube into her waistband, making it a little easier. Then we walked the 10 steps to the kitchen counter, often hand in hand. The fun was over. It was time to get to the business of bedtime.

I helped her lift the tube out from under her pajama shirt and gently elevated both the tube and her hands onto the counter top. Until a few weeks ago, she could do that herself.

While I readied the syringe, Kathy slid her hand along the counter top, over the tube, and folded it in half so that the contents of her stomach wouldn't leak out when the end cap was pulled off. She held the tube shut with her left hand, and with her right hand began to remove the piece of black duct tape that kept the end from popping open.

The little strap of vinyl that had originally held the end cap in place broke a few weeks after she had the tube installed. The replacement cap that we received was twice as big as the original and looked like it would be extremely uncomfortable to tuck into her waistband. So she tossed the new one into a box and decided to fix the old one with a tiny piece of black duct tape.

How can a man not love a woman who can fix things with duct tape? It worked great and each strip of tape could be used over and over for about a week before it needed to be replaced.

For the past couple weeks, though, it had become a challenge for Kathy to get the tape off and pop open the cap. The limited, fine-motor skills of her fingers made it difficult for her to grasp and lift the tiny strip of tape, but she always tried before motioning to me that she'd like some help.

While Kathy worked on opening the feeding tube, I finished preparing the LiverMate. That involved more shaking. On good nights, when we were feeling silly and expecting a good night's sleep, I sometimes danced around the room, shaking the tiny vial as if it were a maraca. It made her laugh. We both needed that.

But bedtime hadn't felt like an occasion for dancing in several weeks. That Tuesday night I simply gave it a few good shakes and opened the lid.

LiverMate has an interesting characteristic: even after I shook it, there were still little particles, like grains of charcoal, floating around and settling to the bottom. It took deft maneuvering with the syringe to capture all of these, and

Kathy was never satisfied until every last one was in her stomach.

Over time I developed a technique of swirling the syringe around the bottom edges of the container as I pulled up on the plunger, chasing down the flighty specks in much the same way that I chased down the goldfish in our pond at the end of the summer.

When it came to LiverMate, I was always in a rush. For some reason if the stuff sat in the syringe for more than about three seconds the plunger would freeze in place and I'd have to start over. That night Kathy got the tape off herself, so I quickly mated the syringe with the tube and passed it off to her to so she could do the pushing. Just as I'd developed a technique for getting all of the little black specks *into* the syringe, she'd figured out a way to make sure that they all came back out. LiverMate, like so many things, was a team effort.

Lately, it had been getting more difficult for her to push down on the syringe. Sometimes I put my hand over hers and we pushed the plunger down together. But she always took the first try alone and usually succeeded.

Then it was off to the bedroom.

Getting settled into bed had been an unpleasant event for months, but after Kathy hurt her neck and shoulders, she'd lost more of her strength and it had become a major challenge.

The number of pillows and their positioning was changed nearly every night. In early October, when she had finally escaped from saliva hell by regulating her salt and potassium intake, she went from five to three pillows.

But the pillow pile was enlarged again the first week of November when she cut back her salt intake because of water retention in her ankles. Within a day of doing that, the saliva again began to flow.

So that Tuesday, to accommodate the saliva as well as her neck and shoulder pain, we once again started building a gigantic nest of pillows. First we placed a wedge pillow on the bottom, followed by an extra-firm pillow near the headboard, followed by three standard pillows layered on top, like shingles.

The only way for Kathy to know if she would be comfortable with that set-up was for her to try it. But getting into bed was no easy task. For one thing, our bed was very high. The extra thick, pillow-top mattress meant that even when she was healthy she practically needed to vault her 5-foot-3-inch body into bed. Now, with very little use of her arms, that vaulting took on a whole new dimension.

She couldn't sleep on her back for fear of choking, which meant that she needed to sleep on her side. Which side had to be predetermined, because the way she got into bed was different if she wanted to end up on her left side than if she wanted to end up on her right side. She usually started out on her right side, facing away from me, because that was a little more comfortable, with the weight off of her left shoulder.

First, she needed to stand alongside the bed and slide up toward the headboard until her butt was even with the bottom pillow. Then she'd literally jump herself up onto the bottom pillow, bend at the waist, and try to land her torso and shoulders onto the higher pillows. It wasn't unlike pictures I've seen of tuna being pulled into a fishing boat. If she overshot, she'd end up on her back with no way to move until I helped sit her back up, ready for a second try. If she didn't jump high enough she risked sliding back down over the edge of the bed onto the floor.

If all went well and she correctly positioned her upper body on the pillows, her feet would still be hanging over the edge, no longer able to touch the ground. She had to push her feet against the wall and night stand in order to get her butt further onto the bed. It usually took two or three good pushes to align her hips with her torso.

Sometimes she'd end up on top of her arm. When that happened she'd either scoot herself back off the bed or thrash her feet until I figured out what was wrong and helped her.

She preferred to do it herself, though.

Once her upper body was in place, she would lift her legs up onto the bed. Years of bicycling had given her very strong legs, and even though she could barely lift them straight up to climb stairs, she could still do a pretty good job of lifting them sideways to get them into bed.

The final step of getting into bed would be a sort of running motion with her feet to try to push herself higher into the pillows, shaping them into a sort of nest around her shoulders.

Only after all of that effort could she tell if the pillows were positioned correctly. Very seldom did we get it right the first try. So she'd scoot herself back to the side of the bed, usually managing to stop herself just before tumbling off the edge.

Back out of bed, she would direct me how to reposition the pillows because her arms weren't strong enough to move them herself. She used hand signals and head shakes until I got the pillows where she thought they should be. Sometimes a pillow would be added. Sometimes one would be taken away. Other times I tore apart the whole pile and started again from scratch, maybe bringing in one of the small pillows from the couch.

Then the whole process would begin anew. It wasn't at all uncommon for this to happen four or five times before she finally got settled into bed.

When she was finally in place to stay, she'd use her knee to kick her hands and arms up toward her face. Then it was my turn again.

I placed a tightly-rolled bath towel between her waist and her chin. This was followed by positioning a loosely folded hand towel between her chin and the end of the rolled-up bath towel. The purpose of the towels was to hold her mouth shut as she slept, which helped solve the problem of her getting a dry mouth.

Finally, I would pull the covers over her in a sort of an L

shape; up over her back and shoulders, but pulled down in the front so that they didn't cover her arms or hands. The weight of the covers, even just the sheets, was more than she could lift, and she'd end up feeling trapped, which she feared more than just about anything.

This whole process usually took about 20 to 30 minutes. Once she was settled into bed, I'd finish getting ready for bed and join her.

Then the real torture began.

Sleep deprivation is outlawed by the Geneva Convention. It is considered a form of torture. I can understand why.

For the past few months, Kathy had been getting up five or six times during the night, usually to use the bathroom, suction her throat or swallow some water. Often, all three on the same trip. Before she'd get back into bed, I'd need to help her pull up her pajama bottoms. She was always concerned about waking me, so she'd quietly come and stand next to my side of the bed so that I could easily reach out and help her without getting up myself.

We had it worked out pretty well. First, she'd face away from me so I could pull up the back, then she'd turn so I could pull up the front and tuck the tube into her waistband. At night, I tried not to pull her pants up very high so that it would be easier for her to get them down on her own in the bathroom.

Once her PJs were in place, she'd go around to the other side of the bed to get back in. If she had been on her left side before she got out of bed, she usually wanted to end up on her right side when she got back in. Each side took an entirely different, but just as difficult, set of gymnastics.

During the night, she usually settled for whatever way the pillows had been positioned when we first went to bed; however it wasn't uncommon for the pillows to shift as she got out of bed and I needed to return them to their original positions before she got back in. As soon as she was in bed, I put the towels back under her chin and covered her.

I got pretty good at putting the covers over her without

getting out of bed. A week earlier I discovered that if I pinned together the sheet, blanket and bedspread, I could cast them out over her as a single unit, like a fishing net. Then all I had to do was move them away from her arms and hands and fall back asleep, until she woke up again, usually in about an hour to an hour and a half.

I'd taken to watching the clock and counting how often she got up. That night it was about every 30 or 40 minutes. About half the time she headed to the bathroom; the other times she would get out of bed in order to turn over.

Around 4:30 a.m. she came back from the bathroom with no pajama bottoms. She hadn't been able to get out of bed quickly enough and ended up wetting herself and the edge of the bed. I put a towel over her side of the bed, and she bounced back in and eventually went back to sleep. She still got up several more times after that for a grand total of 11. Each time getting back in often took several attempts.

Finally, the night's torture ended. It was Wednesday morning.

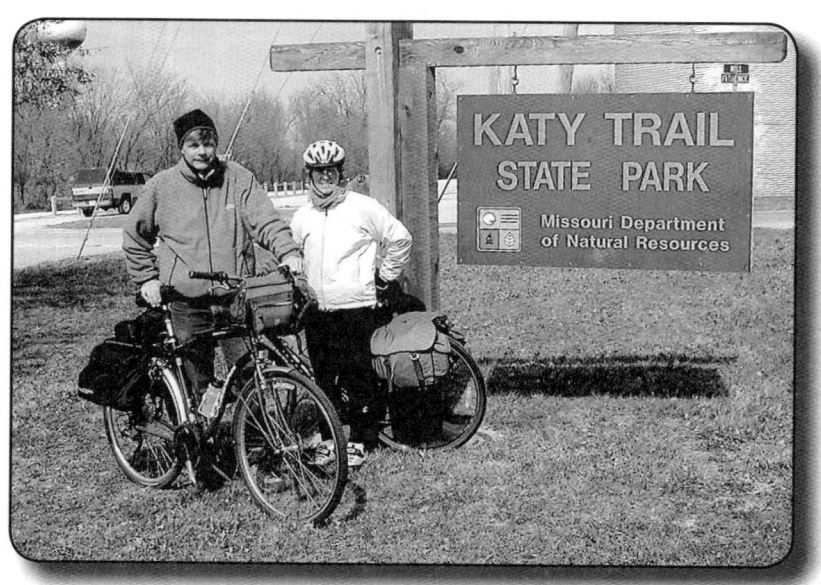

April 2005, ready to bike across Missouri.

CHAPTER SIX
Jasmine Tea & Watermelon

On Wednesday, Nov. 7, 2007, we got up about 7:45, the same time as most days. The difference was that this morning I helped Kathy wash up from her accident the night before. She stood in front of the sink, hands resting on the edge, while I sudsed her up from waist to foot. The fact that she couldn't lift her head gave her an especially defeated look. She didn't say anything about it. Neither did I. There was no need to. We had gotten very good at communicating with each other non-verbally.

Choosing her clothes was both very simple and very difficult. There weren't many clothes that she could wear. Her wardrobe had become limited to a small collection of comfortable shirts and lightweight, oversized pants that could easily be pulled on and off. Because it was getting colder, her most practical and comfortable outfit, a pair of black, jersey shorts that she'd made for herself, and one of her gardening T-shirts, wasn't warm enough, so we turned up the heat a degree.

Her long pants were folded and stacked on a small bench at the foot of the bed. There were only two or three pair that she wore regularly. The other half dozen remained at the bottom of the pile. Most had recently come from the thrift store and were three sizes too big. "I look so frumpy" she wrote on her board. An e-mail to daughter Emily said:

> My clothes r a total mess. I can't wear heavy stuff...evn clothes from last winter don't work anymore. I have so-many nic eclothes that never see the light of day.

I'd been helping her get dressed for months. Each morning we dressed together; it had become as normal to me as getting dressed myself. She picked out her clothes while I put on mine, and then I'd help her get dressed.

Things like her turtleneck shirts (fear of ripping off her ears) and sports bras (fear of ripping off something else) I found quite challenging, but she was good-natured about it, always forgiving my fumbling. Eventually, the troublesome items worked their way out of the rotation.

Up until late October, she sat on the stairs and put on her own shoes, using a soft-handled pliers to pull them on, and patience to tie them. The past few days, though, I helped her with both, unless she decided to wear her Crocs. She always liked those strange rubber clogs. I think that part of the reason they were special to her was because they were a gift from Emily. She also liked them because she could easily slip them on and off by herself, and they still fit fine over her swelling feet.

The swelling in her ankles and feet was new. It only began about a week earlier. We did some quick research and nearly everything we found said that it was most likely water retention, that we should cut back on salt, that she should drink more water, and that it wasn't a serious problem.

Cutting back on salt was a problem, though. We had finally, through trial and error and monitoring of her blood tests, found that with a precise amount of salt and potassium in her diet each day, she could be released from saliva hell. One-and-a-half teaspoons of canning and pickling salt blended into each meal, along with four potassium tablets did the trick. Drop the amount by a quarter teaspoon of salt and the saliva came back. Raise it and the saliva turned thick and sticky.

For the past month and a half, she not only solved the saliva problem, but the sodium and potassium levels in her last blood tests finally rose to the level needed to help her nerves heal. No drooling made it much more comfortable for her to go out in public, too.

Throughout most of the summer, on Saturday mornings we went to the Farmer's Market. Kathy would stay in the car while I quickly visited the stands of the organic farmers. But in late August, when my daughter, Hilary, was visiting, Kathy's saliva was less of a problem and we all went to the market together; a great experience.

That same Saturday Kathy expanded her siphoning experiment and even tried eating some solid food.

We had first tried the siphon idea earlier that week and she was eager to continue using it. This time, we tried Kathy's favorite beverage, organic Jasmine tea.

She sat on the stool at the kitchen counter, as usual, and I held the cup above her head while she directed the tiny stream of tea into her mouth.

Most of it ran back out. The towel on the counter was soaked. The long sleeves of her shirt were soaked. But she was able to swallow some of it!

Jasmine tea was one of the last things that she had drunk before she lost her ability to swallow a year earlier. And now she was drinking some again. I hadn't seen her that happy in months. There was no question that all of her careful work of detoxifying her body and building it up nutritionally was paying off. She was beginning to heal; she was doing the impossible.

After the tea was gone, she tried small pieces of watermelon and fresh raspberries that we'd bought at the market. First, she put a bite-sized piece into her mouth using the tiny fork usually used on the pickle tray. Since she wasn't able to move it around with her tongue, which at that point hadn't had even the slightest movement in about a year, she used her finger to push it around over her teeth. She told me later that she didn't actually swallow any of the melon or raspberries, but that simply enjoying the taste and feel of it in her mouth was an incredible experience. The fact that she didn't choke on any of it made her very hopeful that she' would someday once again be able to eat and drink.

The smile on her face that afternoon was unforgettable. I can still picture her sitting at the counter, sleeves soaking wet, bits of melon clinging to her chin, absolutely thrilled.

Later that afternoon she decided to try taking a nap in the hammock. That had always been one of her favorite spots to read and nap, but because of the saliva causing her to choke when she was on her back, she had been unable to enjoy it all summer. The couple of times that she tried, she needed to get out in a panic after only a few minutes. This time she rested there for almost an hour.

That whole Saturday was fun: Kathy was out with her family; she walked around in public without drooling; she and Hilary planned the next step of a quilting project they were going to do together; she drank jasmine tea; she tasted real food; she slept in the hammock.

This is how Kathy described that Saturday to son Keith and daughter Emily:

> I would consider today a near perfect day I got to lay in the hammock for quite awhile. I tasted watermelon, tea, and raspberries.
>
> I seem to have made a turn around in the saliva. Now my mouth is totally dry and when I rinse the saliva turns to paste. Let's hope this is on the route to swallowing again.
>
> The air today is so sweet...
>
> Hilary was here overnight. ... We went to Farmers Market this morning.
>
> I hope yer days were perfect too.
>
> Love you guys so very much
>
> mom xoxoOO

CHAPTER SEVEN
"I Am Going to Beat This Monster Within Me!"

Kathy's goal for Wednesday, Nov. 7, 2007, was to stop the pain in her neck and help *me* get a good night's sleep.

But that would come later. First, it was time for breakfast.

Breakfast was an adventure in nutrition. It consisted of three hardboiled eggs, an avocado, pistachio granola, hemp seed, cashews, almonds, walnuts, pecans, flax oil, yogurt, a couple of vitamin and mineral supplements and salt. The whole thing was thinned with milk made from one part organic cream and six parts distilled water. That day I added a few fresh cranberries to the mix, too.

This entirely organic mixture was blended together and poured into two one-pint canning jars; one to be used immediately, the other saved for the next morning.

Until mid August, the second pint was saved, then served in the afternoon as the day's fourth meal. But Kathy's metabolism had improved and it had been two and a half months since she needed four meals to sustain her weight and energy.

The two of us listened to Wisconsin Public Radio as she had her breakfast. Our goal was to be finished by 8:50 a.m. That's when Garrison Keillor's "Writer's Almanac" came on. Listening to him drone on about some dead author and recite a poem was something we tried to race ahead of.

Kathy loved a good race. Give her a challenge and she was determined to win.

I remember once, years earlier, when we were on the Sugar River bike trail in southern Wisconsin. We were pedaling along at our usual 12-14 miles per hour when a young biker blew past us like the wind. Kathy decided to take her on.

The young girl noticed that she was being pursued and pedaled even faster. So did Kathy, weaving her way through the other, slower riders on the trail. I tried to keep up, but when my speedometer hit 21 I backed off. Kathy and her rabbit faded off into the distance.

Eventually, I caught up with them. They were stopped along the side of the trail, chatting happily, becoming new best friends. They'd ridden neck and neck for almost five miles. The teenage girl told Kathy that she'd biked over mountain passes with her family and thought that this flat bike trail was pretty lame. She was impressed that an old gal had kept up with her. Kathy told her about her days of cross-country biking, and it turned out they had biked over one of the same mountain passes.

Kathy loved to take on challenges. And even though she'd fight with every ounce of her energy to not lose, she usually made friends in the process.

That's how she approached being diagnosed with ALS. The medical establishment told her that it was a race that could not be won. She was determined to prove them wrong, and in the process she became friends with a whole group of interesting people.

After being diagnosed at the ALS clinic at the University of Wisconsin she wrote on her board in large black letters: "I AM GOING TO BEAT THIS MONSTER WITHIN ME!" Ever since, she'd been battling the monster with all of her might.

Now, though, she needed to win a skirmish: stop the pain in her neck and shoulder so she could get some sleep.

We had a 10 a.m. appointment that Wednesday morning

with Dr. Jodi Swartz, a young chiropractor with a gentle touch and healing spirit. It would be our second visit. Jodi had been recommended by Sarah Pederson, a young massage therapist who would be stopping over to our house later in the day.

Jodi was a great discovery. Before we even met her, Sarah had talked with her about Kathy's situation and helped sensitize her to Kathy's special needs: Sarah had pointed out that Kathy couldn't lie down flat on her back because of choking concerns and that she couldn't lie on her stomach because of the feeding tube. That meant Jodi would need to treat Kathy as she sat in a chair. Sarah also told Jodi about Kathy's neurological problems, so her goal was to not only treat the knot in her neck but also encourage her nervous system to function better.

On our first visit, two days earlier, Jodi ran some electrical tests to determine what nerve action was taking place in Kathy's spine. The upper five vertebrae showed reduced nerve signals. The upper-most vertebra, at the base of her neck, appeared to be under a substantial amount of stress, indicating extremely low function.

There was also a reduced signal at the lowest part of her spine. Jodi speculated that this was most likely caused by Kathy shifting her stance and weight to lesson the pain in her neck, and from lifting with her shoulders to accommodate the weakness in her arms.

The treatment both days involved gently moving the misaligned vertebrae with a small instrument called an activator, followed by stimulating the tissues in her shoulder with an electrical stimulation machine. Kathy especially liked the way that the machine relaxed her muscles and reduced the pain.

We asked Jodi if such a machine was available for home use. Nerve stimulation seemed just the thing for Kathy, and we were already thinking of other places on her body that it could be used. Jodi said that she was sure that small models were available and told us that she'd check to see if any were sold locally.

Kathy felt that the combination of treatments worked well and scheduled another appointment for Friday, optimistic that the pain would eventually cease and that she'd be able to lift her head again.

Jodi suggested that we start putting a rolled-up towel under Kathy's chin during the day to help hold her head up and take some of the strain off of her tender neck muscles. Another option was to buy a soft cervical collar, the sort of thing used for whiplash injuries.

At 11:30 it was time for lunch. Lunch was the same as the previous night's supper. Just as for breakfast, one blender full was enough to fill two pint jars, one for immediate use and the other saved for later, in this case the next lunch. It took a long time to prepare each supper meal from scratch so being able to have enough for the following noon was a big time saver. Time was something that always seemed in short supply.

On Wednesdays, I had to leave at noon to teach my freshman English class. Sarah was scheduled to stop over at 3:30 to give Kathy her massage, which meant Kathy would be home alone for about three and a half hours.

I put on my coat and walked over to kiss her goodbye. The look in her eyes was incredibly sad. "You don't want me to go, do you?" I said, more as a comment than a question.

"I'm scared to be home alone," she wrote.

I made a quick phone call and was able to get someone to cover my class on short notice. I set up my school computer on the dining room table so that I could spend the afternoon with Kathy and grade papers at the same time. It was a nice arrangement.

The people at the university had been very accommodating. At the beginning of the semester my department chair was willing to switch my usual 8 a.m. class for a section that began at 1:25, which allowed me to stay home with Kathy through lunch. The fact that I taught at a laptop campus and half of my classes were online allowed me to teach entirely from home on Mondays and Thursdays.

As I began reading freshman essays, Kathy settled in her rocking chair by the window to do some reading of her own. After only a few minutes she got up to go to the bathroom and get a long drink from the special tube I'd built for her. Then she tried to take a nap on the couch, but couldn't get comfortable. I helped her move all of the pillows to the other end of the couch and she tried again, facing in the other direction. Still not much luck. After a few more minutes it was back to the bathroom. Then back to the rocking chair. Then back on the couch.

I was getting tired just watching her.

At about 3, Kathy asked me to help her move the rocking chair so that it would be ready for Sarah when she arrived a half hour later. We turned it around so that she could look out the window at her gardens as Sarah treated her.

The gardens were nearly done for the season, with only a few yellow and purple mums adding brightness to the browns and evergreens. Still, looking out into the yard helped to relax her.

There was nothing that Kathy enjoyed more than being in her gardens. The past summer had been hard for her. Three years ago she tended two dozen gardens through her Garden Tender business. A year later she had to give up her business and tended only her own gardens. During the summer of 2007, I had been doing some of the gardening work under her careful and loving direction.

As yard work became more difficult for her, she found a way to keep involved by writing articles about gardening for the local newspaper. She submitted her latest, about gardening books to read during the winter, only a couple weeks earlier. It was scheduled to appear in the coming Sunday's paper.

Kathy had also begun taking photographs of her flowers. She had an interest in garden photography for a number of years, but because she was so busy tending to the gardens she didn't have much time to photograph them. As the physical work of gardening became more difficult, photography provided a less strenuous way for her to enjoy her gardens and a new way for her to share their beauty.

She purchased a light-weight digital camera and in the summer of 2006 began taking pictures seriously. Each month she'd post pictures on her web site so family and friends could see what was blooming. By the end of the summer she had several thousand images stored in her computer.

Most of her photos were very close and intimate, taken from the perspective of someone who knew her plants well. Many included miniscule critters with whom she shared her gardens; insects and spiders and frogs no bigger than my thumbnail. Because we used no pesticides or herbicides, Kathy's little garden friends could survive to enjoy the blooms as much as she did.

Most casual viewers of her gardens, myself included, seldom noticed these little critters. Kathy delighted in their company. She always showed me their portraits on her computer, sometimes within minutes of taking them. Other times she'd come in and grab me by the hand, pull me outside and lead me to a particular leaf or flower so that I, too, could meet the new friend she'd just made.

A few minutes after 3:30, Sarah Pederson drove into our driveway. Sarah, in her late 20s, ran Gaia Massage and Yoga in a storefront studio in downtown Eau Claire.

We'd been advised to find someone who could do therapeutic massage and someone who could do acupressure, but we hadn't been having much luck. I began checking out the places listed under "massage" in the yellow pages, but they all seemed to be day spas, where the point of the massage was to make you feel special. That's not what we were looking for. We needed to find someone who did therapeutic massage; someone who could help Kathy heal her body. I also hadn't found anyone who did acupressure, which is similar in philosophy to acupuncture, but doesn't use needles.

At the end of summer, while I was conducting my search

for someone who could do the right kind of massage, Tricia, a friend of Kathy's, stopped over for a visit. Tricia designed the newsletter at the nature center where Kathy worked briefly as assistant director. I was in charge of the nature center's web site until the week before Tricia stopped by.

The previous summer Tricia had a kidney transplant and was very much in tune with the sorts of holistic health approaches that Kathy was using. As they chatted, Kathy mentioned that she was trying to find people who could do acupressure and therapeutic massage.

Tricia knew exactly whom we should contact: Sarah Pederson. Sarah could do both. Not only was Sarah very skilled and intuitive, Tricia said, but she was also a very caring person. So caring, in fact, that Sarah was the person who had donated her kidney to Tricia.

I called Sarah about an hour later, only to discover that she had already received a call from Tricia, who had told her all about Kathy. We scheduled an appointment with Sarah for the next morning.

Sarah and Kathy hit it off instantly. At that time, in late August, we explained to Sarah that we were especially interested in having her work on Kathy's hands. For some time, Kathy's fingers had been curling inwards. It was impossible for her to completely open her hand or have total control of where her fingers went. That made it especially difficult for her to type, which was a problem since one of her main ways of communicating was with the computer keyboard.

I had been massaging Kathy's hands regularly for the past couple months, usually in the evening as we sat on the couch watching TV. It was pleasant—we always loved holding hands—but my efforts didn't really seem to have any effect on her ability to straighten her fingers.

Sarah had a different approach. Instead of working only on the fingers and hands, she worked on the nerve passages all the way from Kathy's elbow to her fingertips. She pressed ever so gently and moved very, very slowly, combining the acupressure and message.

As Kathy was having her first treatment, I decided to walk over to the library to return some books. When I came back an hour later, they were just finishing. Kathy had a very relaxed and satisfied look on her face. She held out her hand, fingers curled up as usual. Then she extended her fingers until her hand was flat. She refolded her fingers and stretched them out again.

I wasn't sure if I should hug Kathy or Sarah. The medical "experts" had told us that with ALS the nerves die and disappear. Sarah's healing touch had just proven that the nerves were still there. They just needed to be stimulated and retrained to function. Another sign of hope.

About an hour after that first treatment, Kathy's fingers were once again curled. But each week it became easier to get them to open. After three appointments, Sarah offered to come to our house. Kathy looked forward to her visits all week.

Because of Kathy's fall in the kitchen, Wednesday's treatment included massaging her neck and shoulders as well as her arms and hands. I sat in the dining room grading papers while she worked. The two chatted, Sarah with her voice and Kathy with her white board. In three months, the two of them had become close friends.

Sarah stayed for about an hour and 15 minutes that day. At the end of the session, the two of them worked out a new schedule: starting next Wednesday, Sarah was going to stop by twice weekly. Kathy wanted Sarah to add the second day to begin working on her facial muscles to prepare her for once again being able to eat.

Have you ever had the feeling that some things are just supposed to happen? That was the case with finding Sarah. Not only was she a perfect match for Kathy's needs, both physically and socially, but the day that we walked into her office Sarah said to me, "Tricia told me that you do web sites and just stopped doing the one at the nature reserve. I need someone to maintain my web site and was wondering if you'd like to barter your web services for Kathy's massages?"

A match made, quite possibly, in heaven.

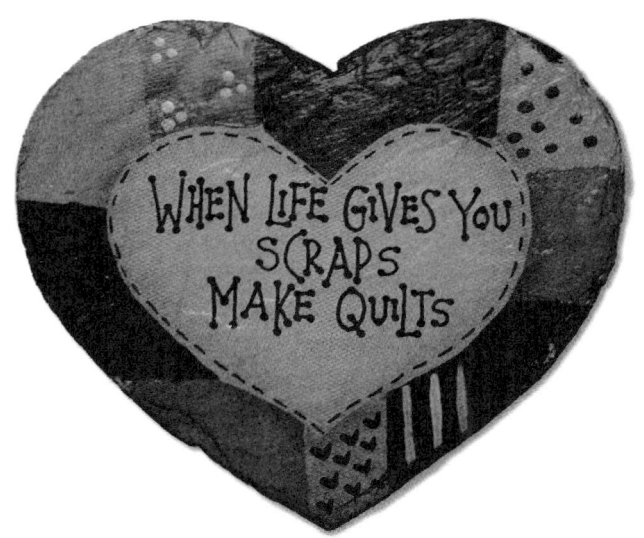

On the wall above Kathy's sewing machine.

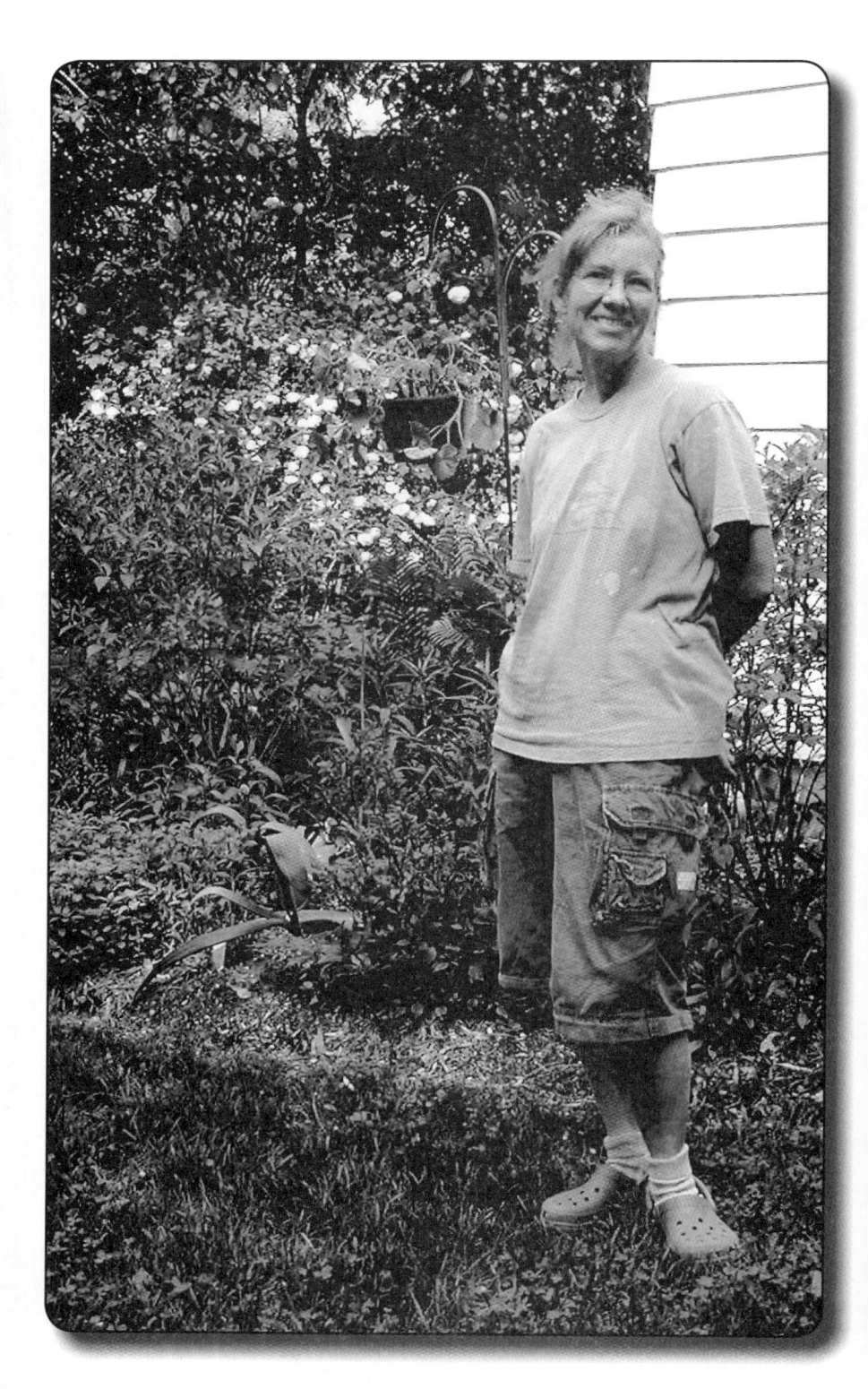

CHAPTER EIGHT
The First Glimmer of Hope

In August of 2006, Kathy came across a reference to the book "Eric is Winning," written by Eric Edney. She immediately requested a copy through inter-library loan. Eric is an ALS survivor who was convinced that the disease is caused by toxins in a person's environment. Rid the body of these toxins and you've got a fighting chance to recover. He was living proof that this thing could be turned around.

As soon as she finished reading the book, she gave it to me. "You need to read this," she wrote. "Then tell me what you think."

It made sense. Besides, we hadn't run across anything else that offered even the slightest bit of hope. It was worth a try.

Kathy had always been concerned about the toxic chemicals in herbicides and pesticides and refused to use them in her gardening business. So that part of Eric's book was preaching to the choir. But Eric went beyond those obvious toxins. He included numerous other household products, including soaps, shampoos, cleaning products, make-up and many pharmaceuticals. He asserted that these products contained chemicals that could damage a person's immune system and nervous system.

The whole point of most of those products was to kill living organisms, in many cases by destroying the nervous system. Many also had the effect of messing with the immune system.

Kathy's nervous system was being destroyed by her immune system. Getting rid of things that could possibly contribute to her demise was a no-brainer. When you have a disease like ALS, any reasonable option is worth trying. This was something that we could easily do ourselves.

We went through our entire house and removed everything that was a possible neurotoxin. We filled several bags with cleaning products, laundry soaps, make-up, shampoos and even air fresheners. Then all of it was discarded and replaced with organic and natural products.

Eric had another assertion. He said that silver amalgam dental fillings contained mercury, which is a known neurotoxin. If you have amalgam fillings in your mouth, you have no chance of recovery because the mercury will continue to leech into your body. He suggested that one of the first things that needed to be done was have them removed.

Most dentists call them silver or amalgam fillings, but they contain 52 percent mercury.

It's pretty common knowledge that mercury is bad for you. Mercury contamination is the reason that we're advised to limit our intake of sea food. The Natural Resources Defense Council says, "Eating fish contaminated with mercury, a poison that interferes with the brain and nervous system, can cause serious health problems."

If you break a thermometer with mercury in it, the vapors from the liquid metal can damage your lungs, kidneys and nervous system. It's against the law for you to put the spilled mercury in a landfill, because it can eventually enter the environment and our food supply. California and many communities have banned the sale of mercury-filled thermometers.

The U.S. Dept. of Health and Human Services sent out an alert about mercury in fish that included, "If you regularly eat types of fish that are high in methylmercury, it can accumulate in your blood stream over time. Methylmercury is removed from the body naturally, but it may take over a year for the levels to drop significantly. Thus, it may be present in a woman even before she becomes pregnant. This is the reason why women who are trying to become pregnant should also avoid eating certain types of fish."

Mercury is nasty stuff. The only place that mercury is considered safe—at least by the American Dental Association—is when it is in your mouth. Go figure.

Kathy had seven mercury fillings, all placed many years earlier. Finding a dentist to remove them was a challenge. Our regular dental office told us that amalgam fillings were completely safe. In fact, a month before we learned about the safety issues of mercury fillings, I'd gone to the dentist because I broke a tooth. He replaced an entire cusp of my back molar with amalgam filling material. I appreciated how quickly and simply he'd fixed my problem, but I had no idea at the time that the material they'd put in my mouth is considered a hazardous and toxic substance in any other setting.

Thanks to the Internet, we discovered a list of dentists who acknowledged the danger of mercury and refused to use it in their offices. One of the dentists listed, Thomas Hebert Jr, was in Eau Claire, where we lived. I scheduled an appointment for Kathy immediately. That was in October of 2006.

Dr. Hebert checked out Kathy's fillings and said that he was willing to try to safely remove them, following something called the Huggins' Protocol. We learned that simply going into a person's mouth and drilling out the mercury fillings can cause more damage than leaving them in. The heat of the drill vaporizes the mercury that is then breathed in by the patient and the dentist. In addition, tiny bits of the toxic filling material can easily be swallowed. If mercury fillings are going to removed, it needs to be done correctly and safely.

Dr. Hebert's other, more immediate, safety concern was Kathy's inability to swallow. The technique that he used would eliminate the worry of breathing mercury or getting it down her throat, but she still needed to be able to swallow her saliva during the process.

Of the seven fillings that Kathy needed removed, six could be replaced with new filling material that was non-toxic to her body, Dr. Hebert recommended a crown for the other tooth. After talking it over, we decided to give it a try.

A few days later Kathy was in the dental chair. They decided to leave the chair upright to help keep Kathy from choking. It didn't work. They were able to replace the amalgam in only one tooth before giving up. It was simply too difficult a procedure to control her saliva and rinse water. She couldn't swallow, but she still had a gag reflex. Dr. Hebert told her she would need to find a different dentist; one who could do it under general anesthesia in a hospital.

We were disappointed, but that didn't seem like it should be all that difficult. We began searching for a different dentist with hospital privileges and in a couple of days found one in town. Fantastic! We scheduled an appointment for later that week to introduce ourselves and explain to the dentist what we needed done.

The first thing we got was the lecture about how amalgam fillings were perfectly safe and there was no reason to remove them. Obviously this woman wasn't on the anti-amalgam list. Nonetheless, we told her that that's what we wanted to do because of Kathy's health situation. The dentist did a very quick exam of Kathy's mouth and said that there were seven fillings and that if she did decide to do the procedure, she would replace all seven with white filling material.

Kathy wrote on her board, "What about putting a crown on one of them?"

"I don't really know how to put this," the dentist said, looking Kathy in the eye, "but you've got Lou Gehrig's disease. What would be the point?"

Then she told us that for ethical reasons she didn't feel that she could do the work. She said it would be unethical for her to remove Kathy's fillings if it was to improve her health.

We came out of there feeling awful. If we had wanted Kathy's fillings removed for cosmetic reasons, there most likely would not have been a problem, but since it was for health reasons it was unethical for her to do the procedure.

As we pulled out of the parking lot, I whipped the bird to the office and said "Asshole!"

Kathy joined in with what little voice she still had, "Dipshit!"

After the dentist's "what's the point?" insult, we wouldn't have let her do the procedure even if she had agreed to do it. We didn't need to surround ourselves with people who saw no hope.

We learned later that the American Dental Association bylaws state that it is unethical for an ADA member to advise a patient that mercury fillings may be unsafe, and a dentist who does so can lose his or her license.

Aargh!

So we searched on. Giving up was not on Kathy's to do list. We contacted a number of anti-mercury dentists within several hours of Eau Claire who were sympathetic to the cause, but all said that they were unable to do the procedure because of Kathy's inability to swallow.

Finally, after several more months, we came upon a dentist who assured us that he could help. But after meeting with him—and paying more than $600 for his initial consultation, some small tooth separators and a full set of impressions of Kathy's teeth—he tried to sell us an untested but very expensive appliance to put in her mouth. It was actually for sleep apnea, but he did his best to convince us that the extra oxygen to Kathy's lungs would be exactly what she needed to fix her problem. He also said that it would strengthen her tongue. And it would only cost $6,000! And guess what? He already had the plaster model of Kathy's teeth, built from the impressions he make during her initial visit, so he could start building the appliance right away.

Not quite what we had in mind.

But he kept calling back to get us to reconsider. He lowered the price to $3,000. We still weren't interested. By then we'd already discarded the worthless tooth separators because they worsened Kathy's saliva problem, making it more likely that she would choke.

His last offer was that he'd do it for the bargain price of $1,500. If it worked, then we could pay the second $1,500. If it didn't, no extra charge.

Finding a dentist to remove Kathy's fillings was turning out to be much more difficult than we expected. We had worked our way through the list of anti-mercury dentists within a reasonable distance, but none of them had hospital privileges to do the procedure under general anesthesia.

A dental assistant in one of the offices we visited commented that a professor at the University of Minnesota dental school taught how to do dentistry while the patient was under general anesthesia. The only problem was, she thought that he'd left the school and she didn't know if he had been replaced.

Only one way to find out. I contacted the dental school and found out that they did, indeed, once again have a professor teaching dental techniques under anesthesia, and that he did, on occasion, see patients.

Finally, some hope!

The soonest that we could see him, though, was in six weeks, at the end of the spring semester. We'd been looking for someone to remove Kathy's mercury fillings for seven months, by then, and had exhausted all other options. We had no other choice. We marked it on the calendar and waited.

During our seven months of searching, Kathy's physical condition continued to go downhill. For example, in 2005 she bicycled more than 3,000 miles during the biking season. In 2006 she started biking as soon as the snow melted and was doing fine and was doing fine, but in June was advised by the ALS specialists to hold back; so she biked only every third or fourth day that summer and ended up riding only about 650 miles for the year.

In the spring of 2007, while we counted down the weeks to our appointment at the dental school, we got out the bikes for our first ride of the season. Hitting the trail together for the first time was an event we looked forward to every spring.

We loaded the bikes into the back of the pickup to avoid pedaling up a steep hill, something we'd begun doing the summer before, and drove down to the Chippewa River Trail, a beautiful, paved bike path less than a mile from our house. The weather was perfect.

There were very few things that Kathy enjoyed more than getting out on her bike. When she was younger, she'd biked across the United States and several sections of Canada. In spite of it being 35 years later, she'd still managed to keep her "biking legs."

At the trail, she stepped onto her bike, put her right leg on the pedal, pushed off and ... crashed.

I jumped off my bike and hurried to see if she way okay. Somehow she managed to keep the tears from flowing. Somehow I did too. The look on her face was pure astonishment. In all of the many thousands of miles that she'd biked, she'd only fallen once before, and that was when she hit an unexpected patch of ice.

I helped untangle her from her bike. She sat in the middle of the trail, stunned, not so much by *what* happened, but *that* it happened. As soon as I knew that she was okay, I picked up her bike and started to take it back to the truck.

She'd have none of it. She was determined to go for a ride and convinced me that if I could help her get started, she'd do fine.

During the previous six months she had lost much of the strength in her arms and, as she just discovered, no longer had the ability to hold the handlebars in place as she pushed off. I helped her up and held the bike upright while she got on. Then I grabbed onto the bike rack and rolled her forward, running beside her like a parent with a child, until she was balanced and moving on her own. Then I hopped on my bike and caught up. As I pedaled along beside her, I could see the strain she was placing on the deteriorating muscles in her arms. It was difficult for her to shift gears, but she was determined to keep going. When we reached the first cross road, she discovered that she barely had the hand strength to apply the brakes.

We biked 12 miles that day. She biked hard and didn't stop until we were back at the truck. I was so proud of her. Her legs were strong; not the least bit tired. But we both knew that was probably the last bike ride we would be taking for awhile. In three years time, Kathy's annual mileage went from 3,000 miles, to 650 miles to 12 miles.

The day before we were scheduled to meet with the dental professor in Minnesota, we got the customary call to confirm our Friday afternoon appointment.

"Yes. We'll be there," I said, looking forward to finally finding someone who could help Kathy remove the toxic fillings from her mouth. Then the receptionist added, "I thought that I should also tell you that the doctor will be leaving the university at the beginning of June."

The beginning of June! I thought. *That was only a few days away.*

"He will still be able to meet with you," the receptionist added, "but he won't be able to actually accept you as a patient to do anything."

My heart sank. I walked into the other room to give Kathy the bad news. We'd run out of options.

Kathy sat quietly, then reached for her board. "Let's go right 2 the source," she wrote. "Let's try 2 find Hal Huggins."

CHAPTER NINE
"Would You Like to Go to Texas?"

We had heard the name Hal Huggins from several of the dentists we talked with. Kathy had also read about his work and knew that he was, literally, the guy who wrote the book on the subject of poisoning from mercury fillings. But how to find him?

Fortunately, we recalled one dentist mentioning that Huggins lived in Colorado Springs. We remembered that because Colorado Springs was where Kathy's daughter, Emily, lived. If we found him and he wanted to talk with us in person, we could stay with Em.

We'd also heard that Hal Huggins was no longer a practicing dentist. In fact, one person said they thought he had lost his license.

That wasn't a problem. We simply wanted to ask his help in locating a dentist in our area. Kathy figured that he probably had lots of contacts, and if anyone could assist us in finding a dentist able to help her, Hal Huggins would be the guy.

I went online and googled "Hal Huggins" and "Colorado Springs." Yes! He had a web site with contact information.

Within a short time, I was on the phone talking to his assistant, Mark, pleading our case. Mark was very polite, asked a number of good questions, and then said. "I'll talk with Dr. Huggins and see if he'll be able to talk with you.

I'll get back to you."

I was hoping for more. "I'll get back to you" sounded too much like another "sorry, we can't help."

About an hour later, the phone rang. It was Mark. "Dr. Huggins will be able to talk with you tomorrow at 1 p.m. for 15 minutes." That was the same time that we were supposed to be meeting with the dental professor at the University of Minnesota. We decided immediately to cancel our U of M appointment.

The next afternoon, I introduced myself to Dr. Huggins and told him about Kathy. Because Kathy couldn't talk, I did all of the phone work and reported back to her what I learned.

Huggins had far more questions for me than I had for him. I told him about the steps that Kathy had already taken to remove the toxins from her body. I explained that in the past nine months, on her own and with the help of an integrative doctor from Wisconsin Dells, she had switched to all organic food; stopped putting any pharmaceutical chemicals into her body; threw out all of our toxic cleaning products and soaps; used only distilled water for drinking and food preparation; and switched to all glass cookware.

He was impressed by her determination to get healthy, in spite of the odds. When I told him that Kathy also refused to let me prepare any of her food in the microwave, he was hooked.

I glanced at my watch. My 15 minutes had stretched past 30, but I had some specific questions that I wanted to ask him. For one thing, he hadn't yet supplied me with the names of any area dentists that we could contact. I also wanted to learn more about him, personally.

I learned that he had been researching and preaching about the toxic effects of dental fillings for nearly four decades. He started out as a practicing dentist and got multiple sclerosis. He wanted to know why, and after serious research determined that it was most likely caused by his regular contact with the mercury that he was putting into people's mouths. He did post-doctorate research in immunology and toxicology and became more and more convinced that mercury from dental fillings and other sources was a major cause of not only MS, but other neuromuscular disorders, including ALS.

Since then, he had worked with more than 3,000 patients. About 1,000 of those had MS; about 300, ALS. As a comparison, our local neurologist had only worked with a couple of ALS patients.

"I've been able to stop the progression or turn around about 30 percent of those ALS cases," Huggins told me. "I'd like to be able to turn around more. Thirty percent is too low."

"Thirty percent is way better than the zero percent at the ALS clinic," I said.

Instead of recommending a nearby dentist, Dr. Huggins invited us to participate in a two-week clinic that he would be conducting in two weeks. He would work with us as a consultant and teacher, and another dentist would remove Kathy's fillings.

The only glitch was that the clinic was going to be held in Texas. Texas is a long way from Wisconsin. No daughter to stay with in Texas. But at this stage, I wasn't about to tell him "nope, too far away."

Then he said something that almost stopped me in my tracks.

"Did you know that I'm also a psychic?"

Oh my god, I thought. *What did I just walk into?*

"I'll bet that I can tell you your wife's weight," he said, reminding me of "The Guesser" at the county fair.

I considered hanging up. I was cautious of encountering people who had a good sales pitch, but were actually trying to take advantage of us. Still, I said, "Okay, how much does she weigh?"

"I believe that she weighs 115 pounds, give or take a pound or two."

I was stunned.

"She weighs 113-pounds-6-ounces," I said. "How did you know that?"

"I'm not a psychic," he laughed. "But nearly every woman I see with ALS weighs within five pounds of 115. I'm not sure why, but I'm working on some theories."

He said that we should let him know soon if we could make it to the Texas clinic. It began in two weeks, and Kathy would need to have both a hair analysis and a special blood test done before we could participate.

I checked my watch as I hung up. My 15 minutes had lasted nearly an hour. My dear, sweet wife, noticing how long I'd been on the phone, was feeling very optimistic, but was quite surprised to hear what I had to report.

"Kathy," I said. "Would you like to go to Texas?"

> Be Peppery, salt of the Earth
> Don't be comfort food.
> NO Tapioca Years!
> Don't go down easily. Stick in someone's craw!
> Be Well-seasoned every season of your life.
> Get Spicier as Time goes On!

Mini-poster designed by Kathy and hung next to her desk. Author of poem unknown.

CHAPTER TEN
Thank God for People Who Step Out of Their Boxes

We had less than two weeks from the time I talked with Hal Huggins on Friday, May 25, 2006, until the time we needed to leave for the clinic in Texas. Thank God for Kathy's practice of making To Do lists. The number of things that we needed to get done to pull this off was a little overwhelming.

Dr. Huggins would be the teacher and dietary consultant during the two-week clinic, but he was not the person who would remove Kathy's fillings. That would be done by Dr. Stuart Nunnally, a dentist from Marble Falls, Texas.

The first thing we needed to do was talk with Dr. Nunnally to see if he would agree to do the procedure. If he said "no," we wouldn't be able to participate in the clinic. Dr. Huggins said that he would contact Nunnally and have him call us.

The day that I talked with Huggins was the Friday of Memorial Day weekend, so I didn't expect a call from Dr. Nunnally's office at least until the following Tuesday.

The very next day, Saturday, Dr. Nunnally himself called, from his home. In a gentle, Texas drawl, he asked a lot of questions, not just about the procedure that we wanted to have done, but about Kathy. I also learned more about him.

Five years earlier, Stuart Nunnally had symptoms of

ALS: he had difficulty walking and had weakness in all of his extremities. When he was referred to an ALS clinic, he decided to contact Dr. Huggins instead.

Nunnally told me that a few weeks before I talked with him, he had completed a triathlon with his daughter. A triathlon consists of swimming, bicycling and running. Five years earlier the man was having difficulty walking, and now he completed a triathlon. I was impressed.

Having experienced the benefits of detoxifying his body, Dr. Nunnally was a true believer. He was living proof that it can work.

He said that he felt sure he could remove Kathy's fillings safely, but that he would need to have a dentist anesthesiologist come to his office.

"We'll set everything up in our office just like in a hospital," he said. "But you will need to talk with the anesthesiologist directly before he decides if he can help you. If he can, you'll need to contract with him for his services." He gave me the number for Lynn Thompson D.D.S., F.A.D.S.A., in Austin. A few days later I talked with Thompson and we worked out all of the details.

Nunnally also asked that we send him Kathy's latest dental X-rays so he could begin planning what he'd be doing, and also so that he could give us an estimate of the cost. He didn't want us to have any surprises when we got to his office in Texas.

He also requested that Kathy submit a blood serum sample for a dental materials compatibility test. He said there are a variety of materials that could be used to replace the mercury fillings in Kathy's mouth, and the compatibility test was to make sure that the material he chose wouldn't cause any reaction in her system.

Those seemed like simple requests.

Tracking down and sending her dental X-rays to Texas was a bit more challenging than expected. We had been carrying one set of X-rays from place to place as we visited different dentists. But the last dentist we'd seen, the guy who wanted to sell us the device for sleep apnea, had taken a more complete and more recent set with digital equipment. Those would be better.

I wasn't overly excited about contacting his office again, but I called and asked that they send Kathy's set of X-rays to Dr. Nunnally. They told me that I would first need to submit a release signed by Kathy and said they'd mail us the form. When I received it a few days later, I immediately mailed it back, assuming that took care of it.

It didn't. It took two more phone calls from me, and a call from Dr. Nunnally's office before they actually sent the X-rays to Texas. Because the X-rays were digital, they were able to send them by e-mail in a matter of seconds. That was pretty slick. But because of all the foot-dragging, the X-rays arrived in Marble Falls the same day that we did. By then, Dr. Nunnally had to make his initial plan of action based on the treatment plan initially put together by Dr. Hebert nine months earlier.

Getting the blood serum for the dental materials compatibility test was an even bigger challenge and almost derailed the whole process. We received a kit that included vials in which to collect and ship the serum; a special mailing container, complete with tiny ice packs; and complete and detailed instructions for the person drawing the blood. It also included a letter requesting the test from a doctor in Colorado, where the actual lab work would be done. All we needed to do was take the kit to our clinic and have them draw a sample of Kathy's blood, spin it down, and put it in their freezer until I came back a few hours later to take it to UPS for overnight delivery.

That didn't seem particularly complicated.

We started with the clinic where Kathy had been a patient for years. They refused to do it. I tried to convince them to change their mind, but they said they couldn't. During the course of our conversation their reason for not doing it varied. First, they said they didn't know how to bill it. I pointed out that Kathy had been in their system for years and her bills had always been paid. Then they told me they thought that there was some new rule from Homeland Security that wouldn't allow me to ship the blood. Finally, they mentioned that the order should have come from one of their doctors. I think that was the honest answer. They didn't want to do the test because it was being requested by someone outside of their usual network.

Since they wouldn't do it, I asked the folks in the clinic's lab if they could suggest another place that would be able to draw the sample. One of them suggested the lab at the hospital where Kathy had her stomach tube placed. She'd be in their system, as well.

A quick phone call ruled out that possibility.

A few blocks from the clinic was a blood plasma center. I stopped in and asked if they could draw and spin down a vial of blood for Kathy. They looked at me as if I were crazy. In spite of the fact that I was standing in a large room, well-staffed and filled with equipment specifically designed for drawing blood, they said that they couldn't help me.

When I got home, Kathy suggested that I call Huggins' office to let them know we weren't having any luck. I talked with Mark. He suggested that I try to find a private lab that did blood testing; the sort of place that a business would use for drug screening. I hadn't even realized that there were private labs that did blood testing.

I found a lab in the area, drove there and talked with the woman in charge. After explaining what I needed and why, she told me that it was possible, however, there was a catch. She could draw the blood only if their own lab did the test. And their lab didn't do the specialized test that we needed.

She suggested that I try the medical clinic or hospital where Kathy usually had her tests done.

Aaaargh!

I don't know if it was the look on my face or divine intervention, but as I turned to walk out the door, the woman said to me, "Come back with your wife Monday morning."

Then she added, "When you get here, don't sign in. I'll do it for you off the books."

Thank God for people who are willing to step outside of their boxes.

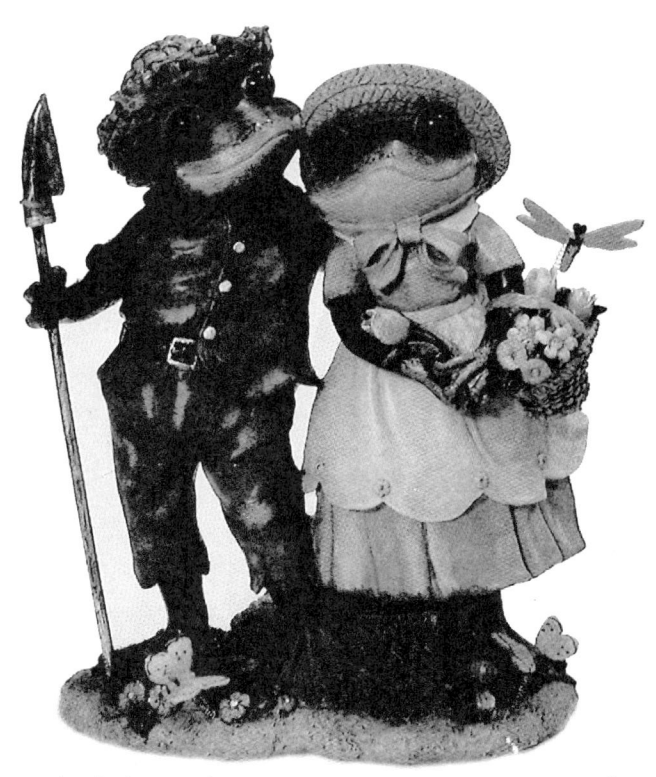

This little garden statue was our anniversary gift to each other the morning that we began our journey to the clinic in Marble Falls, Texas. We thought that it captured the two of us quite nicely.

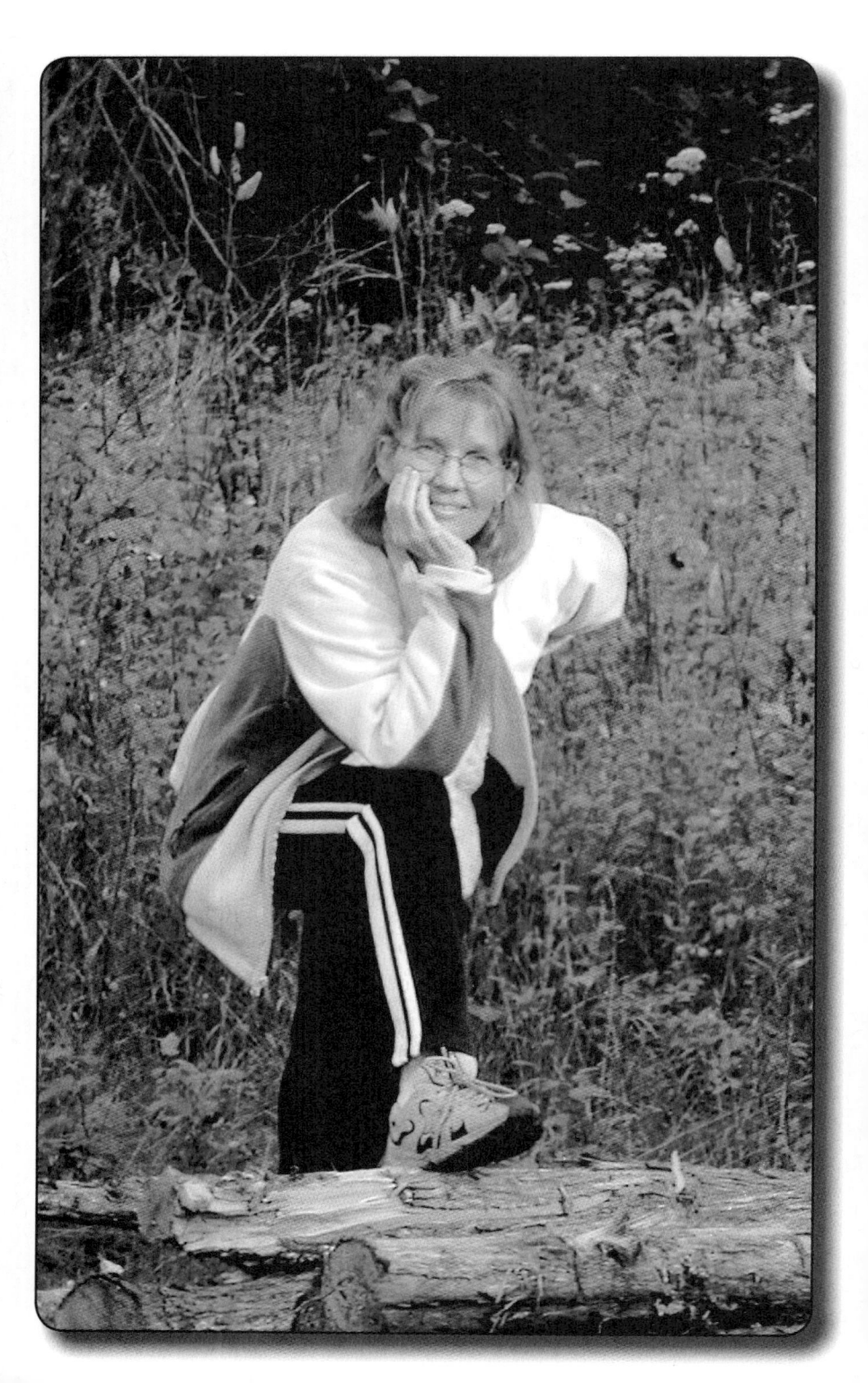

CHAPTER ELEVEN
Getting There is Half the Fun

Besides getting forms, blood and X-rays to Texas, we had to figure out how to get ourselves to Marble Falls. We had done quite a bit of traveling over the years, but with Kathy's nutritional restrictions and the need to always be prepared in case she started choking on her phlegm or saliva, getting from place to place had become much more complicated.

Flying would have been the simplest, but it was essentially out of the question because of her feeding tube. Terror alerts were at their peak then, and the thought of trying to convince the Homeland Security folks to let us board a plane with a cooler of peanut butter jars filled with strange brown and green liquid was daunting. Airlines were even confiscating bottles of shampoo and mouthwash found in carry-on luggage. If they confiscated Kathy's only source of food, we'd be in serious trouble.

Because of our need to stay on a schedule with her meals, trying to pack her food in the checked luggage wouldn't work either. If our checked luggage went to Atlanta while we went to Texas, she would have nothing to eat.

This brought up the question: what would we do for food once we got to Texas? The friendly folks at our local co-op checked their directories to see if Marble Falls had an organic grocery store. Nope. The community did have an organic section in a local supermarket, but we couldn't count on it to have enough of what we'd need for two weeks. The closest organic grocery store was in Austin, 50 miles away.

I sent an e-mail to the local chamber of commerce. They recommended a bison ranch not too far away and also encouraged us to visit the local museum while we were in town.

With no other good options, we decided that we had to drive to Texas and bring all of our food with us. Water, too. We'd been distilling all of our cooking and drinking water for months and had no idea what the quality of the water would be where we'd be staying.

Did I say, "where we'd be staying"? That was another big problem. Because we needed to cook all of Kathy's food from scratch and run it through the blender, and then be able to wash all of the dishes, we needed a place with a kitchen. Rooms were available at the hotel where Dr. Huggins was holding his classes, but they didn't have cooking facilities. A motel with a kitchenette would work, but we couldn't find any in the immediate area.

Then we hit upon the idea of traveling to Texas in a motor home. There was an RV park in the center of Marble Falls, within walking distance of the clinic location. We could simply stay in our home on wheels for the entire trip.

The problem with that idea was that we didn't have a motor home, didn't know anyone who did and none of the local RV dealers had any to rent.

So, with a week to go, we began searching for a small motor home to buy. I visited every RV lot within two hours of Eau Claire. We checked out RVs that were for sale in the classifieds. We even test-drove a couple. They were either too big, too expensive or too run-down.

Finally, a woman from Dr. Nunnally's office came to our rescue. She found a nearby condo, with a full kitchen, that we could rent by the week. I checked it out online, gave them a call and booked it for the two weeks we'd be at the clinic.

"Where to stay" was checked off of Kathy's extensive To

Do list. Kathy's lists kept everything heading in the right direction. She was the most organized person I've ever met and before every trip she wrote out a detailed list of what we needed to accomplish before leaving. With less than two weeks to pull everything together, her lists proved invaluable. As we thought of new things to do or pack, Kathy added them to her lists. As we accomplished a task, she checked it off.

Another item on the list was deciding what we would drive to get to Texas. We had three vehicles to choose from: a 1995 Geo Metro, a 1993 Voyager mini-van with 195,000 miles on it, and a 1998 Dodge Ram pick-up that got only 14 miles per gallon. None of them seemed like a particularly good choice. The Geo was ruled out immediately for being too small. The van would be comfortable and it got pretty good mileage, but it didn't have a working air conditioner and the forecasters were predicting a heat wave.

Ultimately, we decided to pack everything into the covered back of our pick-up. When I say pack everything, I mean everything. We hauled along three coolers and two storage tubs of organic food. We crammed in 15 gallons of distilled water, most of it in glass jars. We even took along a complete set of glass cookware, our own cooking utensils and the soap with which to wash them. Since we had no idea what we might find at the condo, we figured that we needed to play it safe.

Finally, on Friday morning, June 8, 2007, we hit the road, almost exactly a year after our trip to Madison, when we were given the utterly hopeless news that Kathy had ALS and nothing could be done to help her. June 8, 2007, was also our 16th wedding anniversary. I gave Kathy a three-wheeled recumbent bike so she wouldn't have to worry about tipping over, and we could get back out on the trails when we returned from Texas.

For the trip down, we stayed in motels. I pre-made all of the meals for the three-day drive, so all we needed at the motel was a sink with hot water to warm up the jar of food. The week before the trip, I made and blended two meals each time I cooked, one for immediate use, the other to be frozen for the trips down and back, with a couple of spares in case we were delayed. All of her supplements were blended in and each jar was carefully marked with a tag indicating both the intended day and meal.

During the drive, we stopped for lunch at parks and rest areas. That worked fine at first, but the closer we got to Texas, the fewer parks and rest areas we found. A few of our lunch spots were less than esthetically pleasing.

Trying to give Kathy her meals through the feeding tube was awkward in a busy parking lot, such as at a gas station or discount store. So we looked for more private locations, preferably with some shade. One "memorable" location that I selected was the parking lot of an out-of-business Mexican restaurant near Crawford, Texas. It had one small shade tree and I parked under it at just the right angle, so we were somewhat hidden from the nearby traffic.

As I busied myself with setting up Kathy's meal, she was looking more and more frustrated at my choice of location. But I was in a hurry—driving long distances tended to make me feel rushed—so I kept about my business and ignored whatever nonverbal message she was trying to send me.

It wasn't until we were finished and I was looking for a place to dump the rinse water that I noticed what she had been trying to say. Not more than a few yards from the truck, partially hidden by some tall weeds, was the furry, skeletal remains of a skunk. I'd had my back to it the whole time, but from Kathy's vantage point, sitting sideways on the truck seat, facing out the door, the lovely view of the dead skunk was what she got to enjoy all during her meal.

CHAPTER TWELVE
Marble Falls, Texas

Marble Falls, Texas, is 1,431 miles from Eau Claire, Wisconsin. I remember that number because the main road that runs through Marble Falls is Highway 1431. I thought it was pretty cool that when we reached our destination, the highway and the trip odometer both had the same number. Maybe it was a good sign.

The first thing we needed to do was find the condo we'd rented, which was about six miles west of town in a little community called Granite Shoals. After winding our way through an almost rural residential area, we saw the sign: Tropical Hideaway.

The place was perfect for us. We had the whole complex practically to ourselves. When we looked out of our windows we didn't see any of the other units. Instead, we looked out through the trees and cactus to Lake LBJ.

The kitchen was exactly what we needed. There was plenty of counter space on which to organize all of our cooking supplies and a full-sized refrigerator with a large freezer in which to store all of our perishables. By the time I unloaded everything from the truck, it looked as if we had lived there for years.

The clinic didn't officially begin until the following morning, Monday, but we had been instructed to meet at Dr. Nunnally's office on Sunday evening for a short welcome and an overview of what would happen during the next two weeks.

The Nunnally and Freeman dental office was like no other dental office we'd been in. Instead of being bright and cheerful, with rows of matching chairs and a rack of magazines, it was dark and warm. The small waiting area, lit by a mixture of lamps on end tables, felt more like a Victorian dining room than the reception area for a dental clinic. Instead of the standard magazine rack, periodicals were neatly placed on a round, wooden table in the center of the room. The place was very welcoming; classy, without being extravagant.

On the wall was posted a sign:

Drs. Nunnally, Teague & Freeman's View on Mercury Fillings

We strongly oppose the use of mercury filling materials and we recommend the removal of mercury filling materials for the following reasons:

1. Mercury fillings are not stable compounds; mercury is released from these fillings every second for the life of the filling.
2. The United States Environmental Protection Agency, in a report to Congress in December of 1997, stated that the highest body burden of inorganic mercury comes from the release of mercury from amalgam fillings.
3. The World Health Organization has asserted that there is no safe level of mercury exposure.
4. Mercury is considered the most toxic non-radioactive element known to man.
5. Numerous neurological diseases and countless other symptoms are associated with chronic mercury exposure.
6. After removing mercury filling material from a patient's mouth, the dentist is required to store the removed mercury filling in a sealed jar until a hazardous material disposal service can safely dispose of the material.

Our patients should know that our opinion on mercury fillings is in opposition to that of the American Dental Association.

Wow! So much for it being unethical to remove mercury fillings for health reasons. We were in the right place.

We were directed to the conference room with the other people who would be participating in the clinic. There were six participants, each with a caregiver. Attending with a caregiver was a requirement. When I first talked with Dr. Huggins by phone, he said that if you don't have family support, you don't have much of a chance.

He had also pointed out that as the caregiver, I would not only be there to help out with Kathy's physical needs, but I was expected be a full participant in all of the training sessions. We weren't going to be there for a vacation: we were going to be there to begin the process of healing, and that would require total commitment on the part of both of us.

We took our places around the conference room table and were asked to introduce ourselves. None of the participants were from anywhere close to Texas. We thought we had come a long way from Wisconsin, but at 1,431 miles we were the second closest. The others at the clinic were from Michigan, Maine, Oregon, Florida and South Africa.

We had all come for different reasons. Kathy was the only person with ALS. The woman from South Africa had MS and was in a wheelchair. She had difficulty speaking and moving her arms and could barely hold her head up. Her husband said that they exhausted every other option for helping her and, after reading Dr. Huggins' book, "Solving the MS Mystery: Help, Hope and Recovery," decided to come to the United States for the clinic.

On Monday, we met for the blood draw. A nurse from the local hospital came to the dental office and set up shop in the conference room. After all of the problems we had encountered back home trying to get blood drawn, having the nurse come to us was quite a treat.

As we were awaiting Kathy's 9 a.m. turn at the needle, a ruddy-faced older gentleman stuck his head in the door to see what was going on. He made a light-hearted comment to one of the folks in the room, grinned, then slid the door closed behind himself.

"I feel like I just saw the president," said one of the other clinic participants, obviously a star-struck fan.

That was our introduction to Hal Huggins. It was hard to believe that gentle-looking fellow, so admired by one of our fellow participants, could be held in such contempt by the American Dental Association. During the next two weeks we'd learn why, on both counts. Our individual consultation with him wasn't scheduled until Wednesday morning, though, so we needed to wait until then to actually talk with him. All of the dental procedures were handled independently by Dr. Nunnally and his staff.

We were required to begin watching a number of instructional videos about the dangers of dental fillings, the problems with root canals, the harm that can be caused by having teeth pulled improperly, the medical dilemmas caused by the Gulf War and a number of other topics related to poisoning by mercury and other standard dental procedures. We could stop by the clinic any time during the first week to watch the tapes, and we were given a checklist to make sure that we watched them all.

Each person's schedule was slightly different the first week since the dentists needed to complete the dental revision, as they called it, for all of the patients during those first five days. Kathy's revision wasn't scheduled until Thursday.

One of my first care-giver tasks was to make sure that Kathy didn't have anything to eat after 10 the night before her Monday morning blood test. Keeping her from snacking was easy—raiding the cookie jar isn't all that much fun with a feeding tube.

Our main goal in coming to Texas was to get Kathy's fillings removed. We weren't quite sure what to expect during the rest of the two-week clinic. Because we had been so busy arranging for the trip itself, neither of us had time to read any of Huggins' books. We anticipated that he would preach about the dangers of mercury in amalgam fillings. What we would learn during the rest of the two weeks, we weren't sure. But we had driven a long way and were open to anything that would be helpful.

You've probably heard the saying, "False hope is better than no hope at all." We didn't agree with that. We looked at everything critically before deciding what to include in Kathy's treatment plan. False hope was a waste of time and energy. What we did know was that the medical establishment offered Kathy, and other folks with ALS, the "no hope at all" part of the equation. For us, the saying was, "Any hope is better than no hope at all."

Kathy and I had no intention of simply planning for her slow and horrible demise, as we were advised to do by the ALS specialists. So instead of accepting that there was no hope, we searched outside of the system, where we met some people who honestly believed that healing was possible. It wasn't easy to find those folks, but we were beginning to discover that they really did exist.

Stuart Nunnally, D.D.S., was one of those people. He was a true Southern gentleman, polite and soft-spoken with a perpetual smile. Kathy's first appointment with him was Monday morning, shortly after her blood test. He wanted to make sure that everything was in order for her procedure on Thursday. He studied the X-rays his office had received by e-mail. They would work fine. Only a few extra images needed to be taken.

Kathy was nervous when she got into the dental chair. Leaning back caused her to choke on her saliva. Nunnally's calm demeanor quickly put her at ease. He did the exam with her sitting upright.

After inspecting her teeth and fillings, he announced that he was certain he could do the job, do it safely and do it very well. We were glad to hear that, having just spent three days on the road to get there. When it came to the tooth that needed a crown, Nunnally explained that he had chosen a filling material he could easily shape, so he could avoid placing a crown, which would take a second appointment. The filling material he selected was from those listed as least reactive to Kathy's body, based on the blood serum test that we had so much trouble getting done back in Eau Claire.

Nunnally's plan was to remove and replace all seven of Kathy's fillings in one sitting, under general anesthesia. He estimated that it would take about four hours and suggested that while she was under anesthesia, they should also do a complete cleaning. Kathy thought that was a good idea. She had always been faithful about having her teeth cleaned regularly, but the hygienist had been unable to do a decent job the last couple of times because of her choking.

The appointment for Kathy's dental revision was confirmed for Thursday morning, when they were able to coordinate schedules with Dr. Thompson, the dentist anesthesiologist.

The evening before the procedure, Kathy had to come back to the office to have the first of two therapeutic massages. This is the only dental office that I ever heard of that has a massage therapist on staff. The massage was the first step of the process to detoxify Kathy's body. Kathy considered it a treat and asked me to watch closely to see how it was done.

Getting up on the day of Kathy's dental revision was like waking up on Christmas morning. We were both filled with high hopes and grand expectations. While Kathy was a little nervous, she was far more excited. Finally, after nine months of waiting and disappointments, it was actually going to happen.

Just as Dr. Nunnally had told me over the phone, he had one of his procedure rooms set up like an operating room. Dr. Thompson brought along all of the necessary equipment and monitors and everyone was ready to go.

Dr. Nunnally had told Kathy, the day before, that they would do the dental work with her in an upright position so she wouldn't choke, just as he'd done during the examination. But shortly before they put her under, he took me aside and explained that he and Dr. Thompson had decided that once Kathy was anesthetized they would be leaning her back a bit. They felt it was best to not tell her because they didn't want her to panic. But they wanted me to know and understand their plans. I appreciated getting the heads up.

As soon as Kathy was asleep, Dr. Thompson put an oxygen tube through her nose and into her throat. Then he placed a carefully rolled piece of gauze behind her tongue so that there was no possibility that any saliva could obstruct her airway.

Following the protocol developed by Dr. Huggins, readings were taken to determine the positive or negative electrical current coming from each of Kathy's metallic fillings. The fillings would be removed in the order of the charges, beginning with the lowest negative charge to the highest positive charge.

To ensure that no mercury chips got into her mouth as the fillings were removed, a rubber dam was fitted carefully over her mouth and around the selected teeth. It blocked any debris from the old fillings, along with the water sprayed onto her teeth, from getting into her mouth. An ionizer was directed across her body, to help remove any mercury vapor that might escape into the air. For their safety, Dr. Nunnally and his assistant both wore hazmat-type breathing masks so they wouldn't risk inhaling any mercury vapor or particles.

It was quite an operation, to say the least. Every safety precaution was taken for both the patient and the dental crew during the four-hour procedure. During the removal of her fillings, Kathy received intravenous vitamin C, which, Nunnally explained, has been used for decades to aid in detoxifying mercury and other potent toxins.

The next morning we went back for another appointment with Dr. Nunnally, this time to check and adjust Kathy's bite. He spent quite a bit of time doing that, inserting over and over the piece of marking paper between her teeth, to see how they fit together, grinding a little here, a little there, until everything was perfect.

Dr. Nunnally's concern that her bite be perfect gave both Kathy and me a feeling that I still have a hard time describing; it was Hopeful with a capital "H." Why would he bother making certain that Kathy's bite was perfect, if he didn't believe that someday she would once again be using her teeth to chew?!

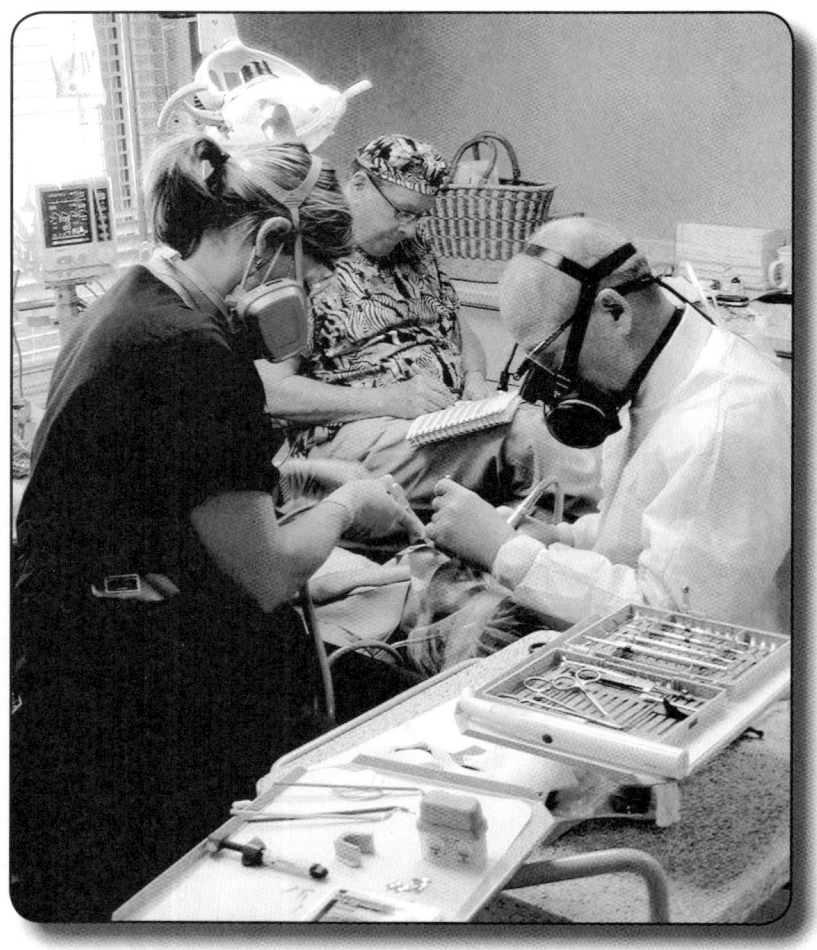

Every safety precaution was used during the removal of Kathy's mercury amalgam dental fillings.

CHAPTER THIRTEEN
Face to Face with Doc Huggins

Our first face-to-face meeting with Hal Huggins, D.D.S., was on Wednesday morning. I had my note pad. Kathy had her Macbook laptop computer. Dr. Huggins had the results of Kathy's tests and her medical history spread out on the table in front of him. Mark, Huggins' assistant, hovered around the edge of the room, ready to assist.

Huggins asked Kathy to tell him her story. He'd already talked with me on the phone, now he wanted to get to know her. Kathy handled her side of the conversation by typing her answers, comments and questions into Sassy, the name she'd given to her laptop speech synthesizer.

In some situations, people would ask Kathy a question, but then look to me for the answer, implying that Kathy was somehow less involved because she couldn't speak. Huggins treated her as a full participant in the discussion.

He understood the need for assistive machines when it came to communication: he was using a special microphone and headset because he was hard of hearing. He got quite a kick out of the fact that, when it came right down to it, Kathy's machine was talking to his machine.

He told us that we would be involved in a much bigger process than simply having Kathy's fillings removed and going home. If healing was going to take place, she and I needed to dedicate everything to the process. It would mean a commitment on the part of both of us.

"There's no such thing as the Huggins' Program," he told us. "What we are going to put together is Kathy's Program, designed specifically for your situation."

"How will we decide which parts of your program to follow?" she asked. We had reached the point we were at in Kathy's health care by using our own filters to accept or reject the advice that was given to us.

"That's simple," he replied with a grin. "Just do everything that I tell you to do."

Kathy had brought along a spreadsheet showing all of the different supplements and vitamins that she was taking. He looked it over quietly, then moved on to the results of her tests.

"You're eating lots of fruit, aren't you?" he said.

"Yes, everyday," she answered proudly, typing her responses into her MacBook and letting it speak her words aloud.

"I've been including several different kinds of fruit in her meals every day," I added. "Mangos, bananas, kiwis, grapes, all organic."

"You have to stop that," he said, handing us each a copy of Kathy's blood test results. "Your glucose levels are too high."

Then he told us about ancestral diets. "Kathy, where are your ancestors from?" he asked.

"Germany," she answered.

"Your body has evolved over time to work best with certain foods, based on where your ancestors are from. Tropical fruits were not part of your ancestors' diets. Your body isn't set up to process them correctly."

I thought about the tub of organic tropical fruits that we'd carefully packed and hauled down from Wisconsin.

"If you were from Hawaii," Huggins continued, "you could probably eat twice as much fruit with no rise in your glucose, because that's what your ancestors would have eaten and that's how your body would have evolved. But you're not from Hawaii. Fruit's out."

A discussion of ancestral diets was not what we were expecting when we signed up to have Kathy's fillings removed. But it made sense.

The blood test results we looked at that morning were extensive. I had never heard of most of them. For example, I had heard of red cell counts and white cell counts, but these tests included numbers for five different kinds of white cells.

Along the left side of the sheet that Huggins handed us were the numbers indicating ranges that he felt were acceptable, followed by a very specific number called the stability point.

The stability point was the number that would be expected of a person in perfect health. Few people ever have those precise numbers in all of the tests, he explained, but his goal for Kathy was that she achieve the stability point for each and every one. She didn't have any room for close enough; she needed to hit the targets precisely. If she could do that, her body would be ready to start healing itself.

He talked to us about each test's results, one by one, pointing out which were acceptable and which were completely off. Quite a few of Kathy's were far off the mark. One, called the albumin level, showed that her body was not at all equipped to build muscle.

Another, called the CPK, was many times too high, an indicator of muscle tissue breakdown.

"You said that you ride your bicycle a lot, right?" he asked. Kathy acknowledged that she did, but now was doing very little. I told him that I'd bought her a three-wheeled recumbent bike so that it would be easier for her to ride, and less dangerous because there was no balancing involved.

"Does it take *any* energy to ride it?" he asked.

"Yes, but not much," said Kathy.

"And how is that energy used? What does it do?"

"It makes the bike go forward."

"Yes!" he said. "I don't want you to use your energy to make your bike go forward, I want you to use your energy to make your healing go forward. No more bicycle riding until your albumin and CPK levels change."

Kathy looked at me with very sad eyes. Once again, she was being told to give up doing what she loved most.

"That's what the doctors at the ALS clinic told us," I said, "and we don't think they were right."

"Well, not stressing your muscles when they can't be rebuilt may be the only thing that those people and I agree on," said Huggins. "You can ride again next year, when your albumin and CPK levels have changed and you've built back your muscles."

We also looked at Kathy's potassium and sodium levels, which are essential to proper nerve transmission. Huggins said he has regularly noticed that the potassium levels of people with ALS are very low. Kathy's potassium and sodium were both way down.

He was especially concerned about Kathy's white blood cells. By comparing the numbers of the five different types of white blood cells he had tested, he explained that, for all practical purposes, Kathy's immune system was no longer functioning. It had essentially done all that it could, lost the battle and had given up.

"That can all be turned around," he said. "I can't cure you, but I can help you change your body chemistries so that your body is able to heal itself."

We had originally thought of Hal Huggins as a dentist on a crusade against mercury fillings. We were quickly coming to realize that his true passion was biochemistry and the way that elements fit together to keep the body healthy. Mercury toxicity was one part of a much bigger puzzle; a puzzle that he was going to help us put back together.

At the conclusion of our first visit, he told us to make some additional changes to Kathy's diet. He'd already eliminated the fruit. Now he told us to stop using milk to thin her meals because of the hormones it contained. I pictured myself sadly pouring out five glass bottles of organic milk that we so carefully trucked along from America's dairyland. But he wasn't anti dairy. We were supposed to start adding butter to her diet—a stick a day—and a teaspoon of canning salt. Before we left, he gave us some minerals and vitamins and said that I should start blending them into Kathy's meals immediately.

The second week of the clinic was, essentially, a course in biochemistry, taught by Dr. Huggins. The purpose was to help us understand the reasons for the dietary changes and to learn how to read the blood tests so we could monitor our progress. Near the end of the week, Kathy had more blood drawn and on the last day we had our final consultation with Dr. Huggins.

In the course of 10 days, some of the numbers were already beginning to improve. Some of this change could have been Kathy's body's response to the dental revision. Part of it may have been caused by the dietary changes and vitamin C infusions. Whatever the reason, it was great to see that it was possible to do something to change Kathy's body chemistry for the better.

There were a lot of numbers on Kathy's blood test list and most of them had a long way to go before they reached their stability points. Still, when we left Texas, we knew what we were shooting for, and we felt like we finally had the ammunition to hit the targets.

We had hope!

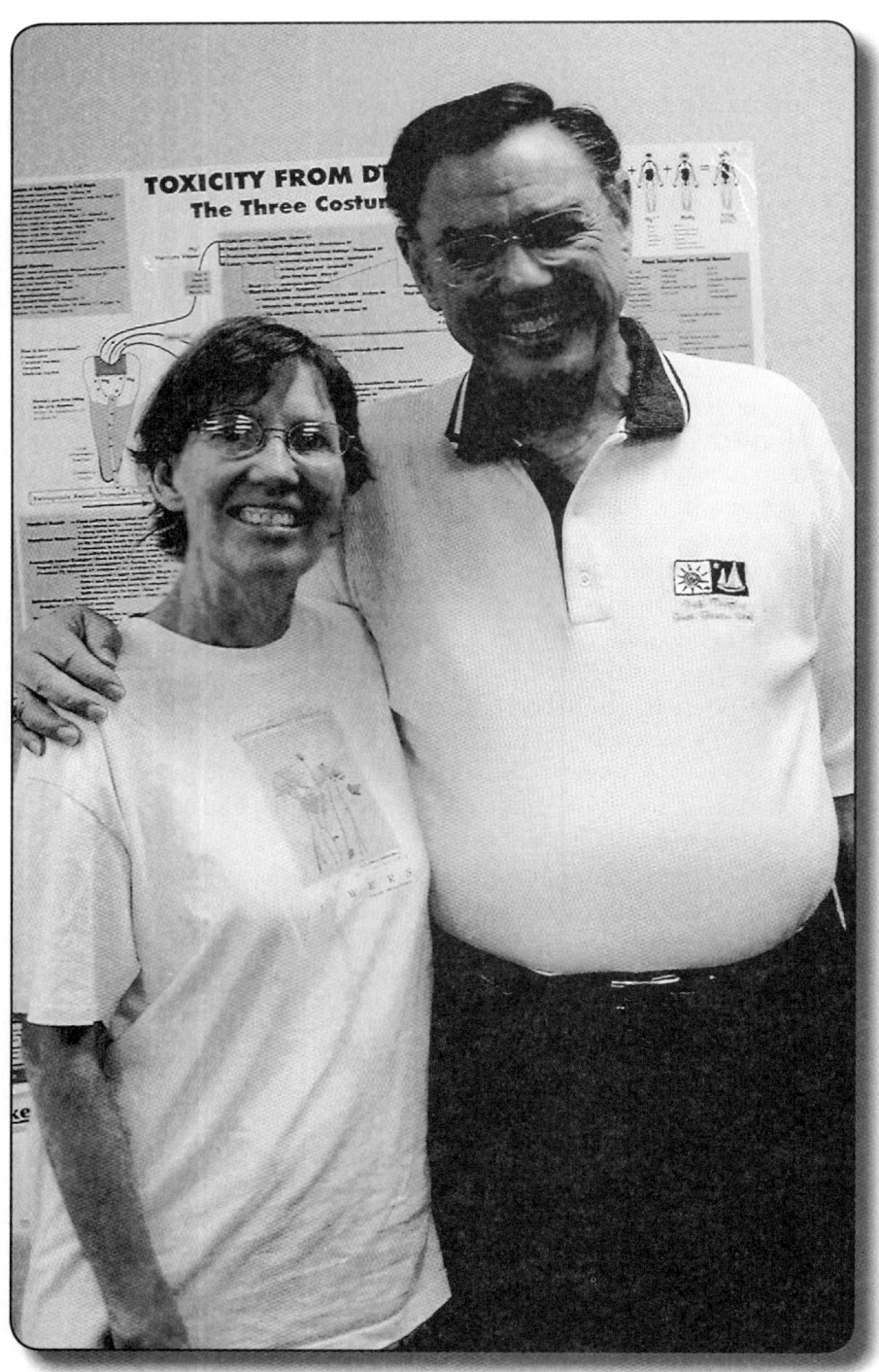
Kathy and Doc Huggins shortly before leaving the clinic in Texas.

CHAPTER FOURTEEN
Let the Healing Begin

It was Wednesday, Nov. 7, 2007, and I was washing the supper dishes.

While I was scrubbing away, I could hear Kathy in the living room on the humping machine. It was actually a Nordic Rider, an exercise machine designed to simultaneously strengthen your arms and legs. We called it a humper because of the way a person looked when using it. Last winter we had it in the basement, where we'd also rigged up a system of trapeze bars, made with ropes and springs, that Kathy used to get some low-impact, winter exercise.

In early October, we decided to bring it upstairs where it would be handier, since it had gotten more difficult for Kathy to go up and down the stairs.

Kathy kept very good records. The previous winter she tracked all of the calisthenics she was doing, including the date and the number of repetitions. It was a long list and included 24 different exercises. She stopped the exercises after Doc Huggins pointed out that her body wasn't yet capable of rebuilding muscle.

Throughout the summer and early fall of 2007, instead of exercises, we went for walks along our country road, usually about a mile or two at a time.

At the beginning of September, the albumin level in her blood tests was at the stability point for the second month in a row. It had reached that level much quicker than would usually be expected. Based on the blood tests, her body was ready to begin building muscle.

That evening she send the following e-mail to her kids:

> Dearest Darlings,
>
> I made it! Got permission 2day 2 start rebuilding muscle. I also requested a pep talk and got a good one. And Hal greeted us 2day as his favorite couple. So things r a lot less discouraging 2day.
>
> Hope everything is jusst dandy 4 u gguys.
>
> Loving u, mom x oOOox

She was thrilled and set up a new, much simpler exercise routine. To ensure that she wouldn't overdo it, we found some very light weights and she reduced her routine from 24 exercises to 10, some modified to accommodate her inability to raise her arms very high. For example, in February she did bicep curls with four-pound weights; two sets of eight repetitions. For her new routine she used a two-pound weight and lifted it straight up and down about a foot off the floor; two sets of 10 repetitions.

When she stopped using the humper in late spring, she had been doing 20 repetitions with her arms in a position to strengthen her biceps and 20 to build up her triceps. When she started again at the end of September, she knocked that down to 15 each. By the second week of October she felt strong enough to go back to 20, which is the number she did that Wednesday, Nov. 7, 2007, while I washed dishes.

I was amazed at her commitment to getting healthy and the strength that she still had and was regaining. I had trouble doing 20 reps on the humper, and she was doing twice that many without getting winded. She was feeling great about once again being able to exercise and thrilled that she could actually do it.

Kathy was doing her best to keep her muscles from atrophying and was especially concerned that her legs had gotten weaker since she's stopped exercising. She was optimistic about building them up again, however rebuilding her muscles and restoring the nerve connections between her brain and her legs were two different challenges.

We were both fascinated and frustrated by the fact that she could push down hard with her legs on the exercise machine, but when she tried to tell those same legs to climb the stairs, it was like her body was in slow motion.

Late in the summer I began helping her up the stairs when I was around. I made a fist and put my hand under her butt like a bike seat, something she was very accustomed to, then walked behind her to provide a bit of a boost. It worked pretty well and she moved up the steps at a steady pace. We weren't sure why that worked. Maybe it was mimicking the sensation of pushing down on the bike pedals. Maybe that little extra boost was all she needed. Maybe it was the confidence she gained by having me close at hand in case she slipped.

The first few days of November, I noticed that she'd started using her laptop downstairs to check her e-mail, rather than ask me to help her up the stairs to her office. I wasn't sure if it was because she didn't want to bother me, or because she was getting too tired to climb the stairs. Either way, she was spending more time downstairs and less time in her office; more time in our shared space and less time in her own space.

After I finished washing the dishes, I hooked up the TV to the stereo so we could hear the country music awards show from bathroom. On Sunday and Wednesday nights, Kathy would soak in a tub of hot water mixed with Epsom salt to help detoxify her system. She'd never been the tub-soaking type, and where some folks find a hot soak relaxing, Kathy always disliked it. Like so many other things, she did it now because she was determined to rid her body of the neurotoxins that were poisoning her.

I started filling the tub, added two cups of Epsom salt,

then helped her undress. When the water was about eight inches deep and 100 degrees, I helped her into the tub. Then I heated the water up to precisely 104. We kept careful track of the temperature with a special thermometer she had for monitoring the heat in her compost bin. We got a kick out of this new use for it.

As soon as the temperature reached 104, she lay back and I covered her up to her neck with a large, wet, beach towel which held in all of the heat. After only a couple of minutes she was ready to get out.

Getting Kathy out of the tub was a much bigger challenge than getting her in. For one thing, she'd be as limp as the towel that covered her. Plus, the tub was unusually narrow, making it difficult for her to get much side-to-side movement. Add to that, the fact that she didn't have much arm strength to help pull herself up—and the fact that I didn't have the arm strength to simply lift her—and getting Kathy out of the tub was a comedy of errors.

"Ready? Move your right leg up under your left leg... okay... good... no... how about you slide to your left... no... can you turn towards the wall? ... okay... good... a little further... now grab the bar with your right hand... no, no, wait, that won't work, then your arms will be crossed when you stand... okay... that's good... try to stand... now, let me get my arms around... geez, you're slippery when you're wet."

One evening, after a few too many nights of my clumsiness, I noticed Kathy sitting on the living room floor next to the couch, slowly moving her legs under herself and getting onto her knees. She was figuring out a method of her own for getting out of the tub. The next time she needed to get out of the bathtub, she showed me exactly how it should be done.

The first step was for me to help her sit up, with her legs folded under her. I joked that she looked like the statue of the little mermaid. Then she shifted her weight up and onto her knees. She was used to getting up from her knees. She'd done it a million times while gardening. She felt confident in that position. Then I helped her slide her right foot forward until it was next to her left knee. Finally, I helped position her hands on the grab bar a few inches above the tub.

From that position, it was a matter of me putting my forearms under her armpits and with a "ready, set, stand," she was up, ready for me to help her out of the tub and into my waiting arms. Planning and teamwork. We could solve darn near anything that way.

Once she was out of the tub we scurried hand-in-hand to her bathroom, hoping that no one had dropped by to catch us rushing through the house naked. The tub was in my bathroom, but we moved to her bathroom because the shower there was better and because the things she needed after her shower were in that room.

As soon as she stepped into her shower, which we set at a cooler-than-normal temperature, I quickly scrubbed her entire body with a loofah sponge. The goal was to wash away any toxins that came out of her pores during the hot bath.

When we were finished, the towels and sponge were immediately tossed into the washing machine so that we didn't risk recontaminating our bodies with whatever she may have sweated out. Did that seem a bit excessive? Sure. But when you're battling a disease as devastating as ALS, "good enough" cannot be part of your vocabulary.

That Wednesday evening we scheduled Kathy's bath a little earlier than usual. Ann would be coming over in a few minutes for a slumber party.

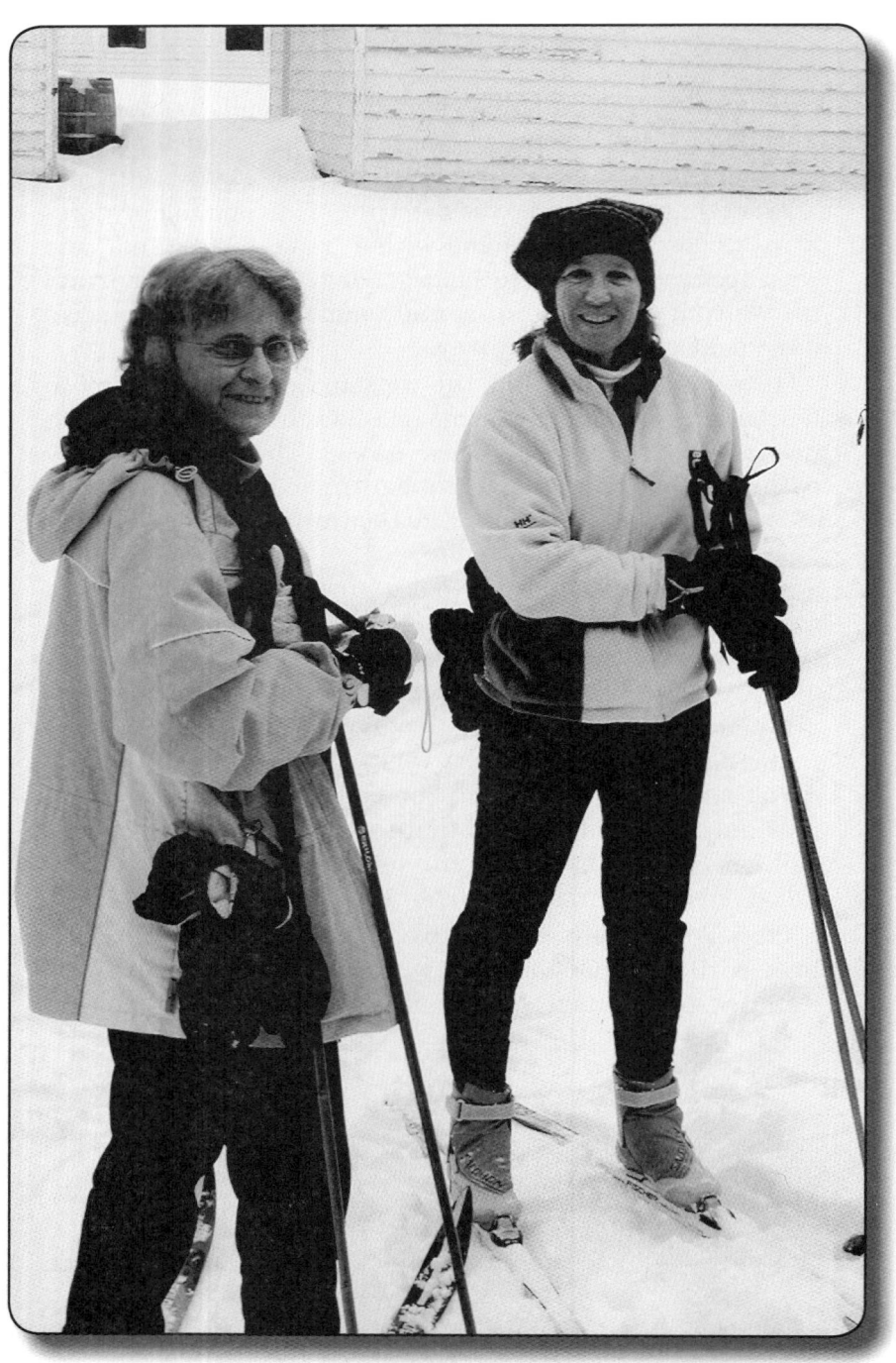

Ann and Kathy in January 2006, following an afternoon
of cross-country skiing along Lake Superior.

CHAPTER FIFTEEN
The Supreme Sacrifice

On Monday, Kathy cryptically wrote, "Ann is going 2 give the supreme sacrifice on Wednesday."

She let me ponder that for a moment, a grin on her face.

"Okay," I said. "I don't have a clue what that means."

"Ann is going 2 come over Wed. nite so U can sleep."

I wasn't getting much more sleep than Kathy, and she could tell that it was taking its toll on me, as well as on her. She knew I was extremely sleep deprived.

"U cuss when U R really tired," Kathy wrote. "U've been cussing a lot lately."

It hadn't occurred to me that while I was working in the kitchen, she was in the living room listening to me muttering obscenities every time I made the slightest blunder. Something as simple as dropping a spoon on the floor had become an "Oh shit!" moment.

She was right. If I was going to be of much use to her, I needed to get some sleep. I was aware of the problem, too, but didn't know what to do about it.

A few days earlier, in an e-mail to my brother, I wrote,

> I can see why they use sleep deprivation as a tool of torture. I'm about ready to confess to anything.

The week before that, I told him,

> Basically, we're just slogging along each day as best as we
> can... lack of sleep has become a big issue. A good night
> is getting up only five or six times... . Some nights it's been
> 11 or 12.

Apparently my lack of sleep was obvious to Ann, as well. She'd volunteered to spend the night with Kathy so that I could get some sleep in the guest room. Kathy considered it a supreme sacrifice for someone to have to sleep with her. I didn't agree with that, but I did have to admit that I was seriously in need of rest.

After her accident the night before, I could tell that Kathy was apprehensive about having someone other than me share her bed. But she desperately wanted me to get a good night's sleep. If she got up 11 times during the night, that meant that I was also awake 11 times. Each time she got out of bed, I helped her get uncovered. If she went to the bathroom, I helped pull up her pants when she returned. After she got back into bed, it was my job to re-cover her. I didn't mind doing these things, but we both realized that this couldn't go on much longer. We needed to get some rest.

Ann stopped in about 9:30, carrying her PJ bag like a kid coming for a sleep over. She appeared ready for what lay ahead.

I wasn't.

What had seemed like a good idea on Monday, now seemed all wrong. My place was beside Kathy, not upstairs in the guest room. I'd rather be tired than have her get an even worse night's sleep because she was in inexperienced hands.

I didn't feel any better when Ann cautioned Kathy that she snored. Kathy had never been able to put up with my snoring; how could she possibly get any sleep with the snoring of a stranger?

Once we handled a few niceties, we needed to explain to Ann what she should expect and what she should do. We warned her that this wasn't going to be a typical sleep over.

Bedtime chatting and giggling had ceased quite some time ago.

Step one, of course, was getting Kathy settled into bed. That was never a quick process, but it took an unusually long time that night to get Kathy's nest of pillows situated correctly. In the process, I showed Ann how to recognize when Kathy needed help getting the covers off so that she could to get out of bed and how to reposition the covers when Kathy returned.

In the past weeks, it had grown increasing common for Kathy to feel trapped under the covers. She would panic and begin kicking in an attempt to escape. My goal was to recognize a potential problem before it happened. If I noticed her having even the slightest problem getting the covers off, I needed to pull the covers out of the way immediately. It was most likely my slow response the night before that caused her to wet the bed, a detail we left out of Ann's training.

It was about 11 by the time Kathy was finally situated in bed as comfortable as she could get. Her shoulder felt better following her chiropractic treatment earlier in the day, but by evening it was again causing a great deal of pain, especially when she tried to lie down.

It was time for me to go upstairs to the guest room. I told Ann to come and get me if she needed any help. "We'll do fine," she said, but the look in her eyes made me wonder if she was now thinking she'd gotten herself into more than she'd planned. "Go upstairs and get some sleep," she said.

It felt so very wrong for me to leave. I gave Kathy a good night kiss and told her I loved her. She looked directly into my eyes and without speaking or writing a word told me, "I'll be okay. Get some sleep."

Instead of feeling excited about getting to sleep alone, I felt as if I'd been banished. I wasn't where I belonged. A stupid feeling, to be sure, but I had a hard time relaxing and woke up every 30 or 40 minutes, the same as always.

At about 2 a.m. I heard the sound of the suction machine

in the bathroom and was almost out of bed and downstairs before I thought, *No, David. Ann is here to take care of her tonight. If she needs you, she'll come and get you.*

I lay still, waiting to hear Ann's feet on the stairway.

Nothing.

No one knocked on my door.

The house fell once again quiet.

I fell back asleep and the next thing I knew it was 7:45 a.m. I'd slept nearly six hours uninterrupted. It had been months since that had happened.

Kathy told me the next evening that I hadn't cussed once all day.

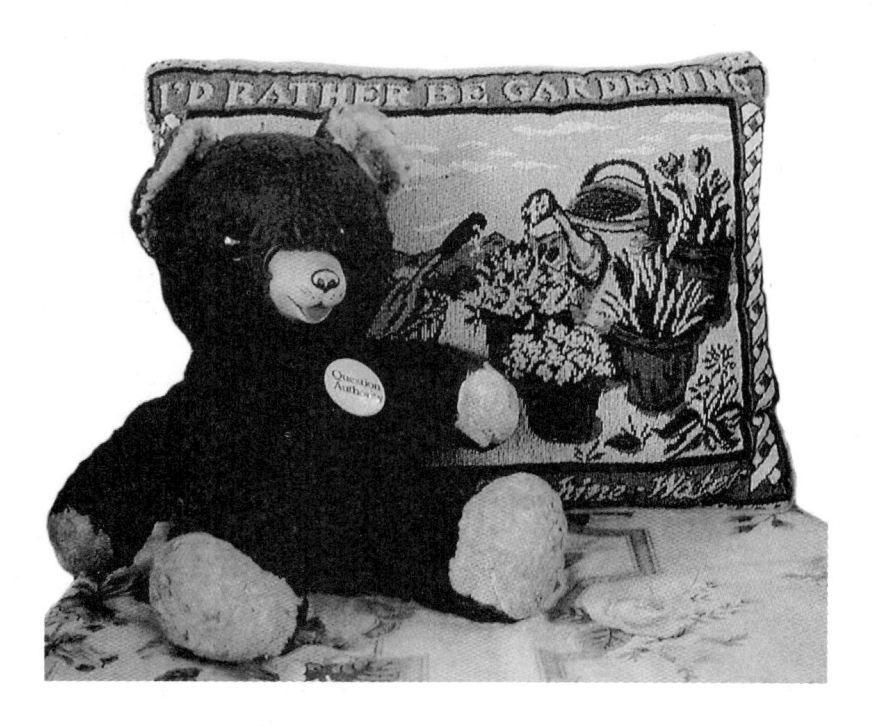

CHAPTER SIXTEEN
Back to the Big Leagues

On Thursday morning, Nov. 8, 2007, I came down from the guest room at about 8. Ann was already dressed, resting on the couch in the living room. I had told her the evening before that we would be on a tight schedule in the morning. She didn't say much about the night before other than that Kathy had gotten up about six times, that it went okay and that she was willing to do it again. She looked tired. I felt a bit guilty having finally gotten some sleep at her expense. But I appreciated it.

On the surface, it looked like the night was a success. Kathy got up only about half as many times as the previous night, and had no accidents.

Unfortunately, even though she didn't get out of bed very often, she told me that she had barely slept. It wasn't easy for her to be in bed with a stranger. She felt like she had to be on her best behavior and not cause too much trouble. Plus, she was very concerned about the possibility of having another accident as had happened the night before.

I appeared to be the only one who benefited from the slumber party. The reason Kathy agreed to the experiment, however, was to help *me* get some rest and she was happy to hear that I'd been able to sleep. I knew that I'd never be willing to do that again, though.

That morning we had an appointment to meet Dr. Carleen Sterner, who we hoped could become our local conduit to the health care network.

It had become obvious in the past weeks that we needed to find someone who could stay with Kathy while I was at work. Ann and Kathy's son, Keith, were handling that much of the time, but it wasn't fair to them to expect they would be with Kathy whenever I was gone. There were home health care organizations in town that could assist us when needed, but I discovered that in order to get their service, it had to be prescribed by a physician.

That was the clinker.

In order to get home health care service, a physician had to authorize it. That was the only way that the insurance company or Medicare would even consider assisting with the cost, and at nearly $25 per hour, cost was a consideration we couldn't disregard.

Nearly everything else we were doing came out of our own pockets. We thought that maybe, for a change, we could get a better return on the insurance premiums we'd been paying over the years.

But Kathy no longer had a local physician. She'd lost all confidence in the physicians she saw early in her illness. We were convinced that their misdiagnoses and long-term prescriptions for short-term medications had most likely aggravated or even helped cause her disease.

The local neurologist we had worked with most recently and closely was a decent guy. Even though he had taken us down the wrong path when he diagnosed Kathy as having myasthenia gravis, we still believed that he had her best interest at heart. He always treated her as a person, not a patient. Unfortunately, a few months earlier, he had to close his practice because of his own health problems.

Besides finding a conduit to the home health care network, we were also looking for someone who could set Kathy up with intravenous vitamin C treatments. Kathy had that treatment twice in Texas and felt that it was helpful and had no bad side effects. Since then, she had been taking vitamin C blended into her meals, but the detoxifying effect would be greater if it was administered intravenously.

Dr. Waters, an integrative health care doctor that we'd seen periodically for the past year, was willing to help, but he was more than two hours away. With winter approaching, we wanted to find someone who could do it locally, preferably in our home. Each treatment took about three hours, so it would work much better where Kathy had easy access to her bathroom, water and suction machine.

We concluded that we had no choice but to find a "real" doctor in town. The trick was to find a doctor who would respect the approach we'd taken to deal with Kathy's disease. We didn't want to be lectured about the worthlessness of what we were doing.

I had been buying organic bath soap at a little store called B Natural, and it occurred to me to ask the owner, a natural medicine consultant, if she knew of any MDs in town who would be sympathetic to our cause. She did. In fact, she had the name and phone number of Carleen Sterner pinned to her bulletin board.

As soon as I got home, I called to make an appointment. We were scheduled for Thursday, Nov. 8, 2007, at 9:30 a.m.

It was now that Thursday morning and we had less than an hour to get dressed, have breakfast and be on our way.

By the time we left for the clinic to meet Dr. Sterner, Kathy was already exhausted. We pulled into the parking lot a few minutes before 9:30. I had a handicap parking permit, so we parked in the handicapped spot closest to the door. It was still about 40 yards to the entrance and by the time we got to the lobby, Kathy was nearly out of energy. She didn't stumble or trip as she walked, which is common with ALS, she was just too tired to go on.

I noticed a row of wheelchairs lined up near the gigantic revolving doors. "Should we try one?" I asked, not sure what her answer would be or if I should even raise the question.

About a month earlier I had come across a wheelchair in good condition at Hope Gospel Mission Bargain Center, an exceptional resale store where we had found most of our glass cookware. The wheelchair was in great shape and cost only $39.

I mentioned it to Kathy. She was annoyed at me for even thinking about it. "U haf 2 ncourage me 2 keep trying," she wrote. "Don't make things easy!"

That morning at the clinic, she was ready for easy.

It was a little unnerving once again being inside a huge medical center. The clinic with which Dr. Sterner was affiliated was attached to Luther Hospital, part of the Mayo Health System. It had been almost a year and a half since we'd sought medical care for Kathy within the "official" health care system. All of our contacts since then had been with individuals in small, personable offices; places where we were welcomed by name when we walked in the door. Compared to what we had gotten used to, this place was huge and intimidating.

Dr. Sterner was part of the women's and family health clinic on the second floor. As the elevator doors opened, I realized that I didn't know if I should push the wheelchair in ahead of me or if I should turn it around and pull it in after me. I chose the latter while some kind folks already in the elevator kept the door from closing.

The wheelchair was as new to Kathy as it was to me. We tried one only once before, about six weeks earlier. We were running errands together and as we walked into Shopko, Kathy noticed an electric shopping cart near the door. As usual, we were in a hurry and even though she was walking fine, she wasn't able to walk fast. She motioned toward the electric cart and gave me a "let's try it" look. I could tell by her expression that she thought it might be fun. She had once terrorized a golf course in a golf cart, so I could only imagine what she'd be like in that powered shopping cart.

She sat down on the seat and pushed a lever that seemed like it should make the cart move. Nothing happened. She tried again. Still nothing. Maybe her hands weren't strong enough to hold the lever all the way down. I tried it. Nothing happened when I held it down, either. I searched for an on and off switch with no luck.

About that time, a clerk walked by and told us that the cart didn't work. "There's a better one plugged in at the other entrance," he said, pointing across the store. "Or you could use that." He nodded toward an old, somewhat battered wheelchair that was pushed under the nearest checkout lane.

"What do you think?" I asked Kathy.

She didn't want to walk across the store to get the other powered cart, so she agreed to try the wheelchair. We scooted through the store in no time. I may have taken a couple of corners a little too quickly and we caught the bottom of a display with the footrest, but that was okay. We hadn't tried anything new for quite awhile. For a few minutes we were having a spontaneous adventure. We had fun.

The wheelchair ride at the hospital that Thursday morning was not as enjoyable.

We checked in at the desk and waited to be called. Kathy's head was hanging low. When they called us, I wheeled her down the hallway. We parked the chair in the corridor and together walked into the examination room.

As always seems to happen first in a medical clinic, the nurse took Kathy's pulse and blood pressure. Even though she was getting monthly blood tests, she had not had her blood pressure taken since June. I was especially interested to see what it would be. A year earlier, almost to the day, her blood pressure was her usual 120 over 74. At that time, I was adding no salt to her meals. Since June, she'd increased her intake of salt considerably. For the past six weeks her diet had included four-and-a-half teaspoons of salt a day, many times the FDA's recommended amount. Conventional wisdom said that her blood pressure should now be much higher. Wrong. It was 120 over 70, slightly less than usual. So much for conventional wisdom.

After waiting a few minutes in the examination room, we were greeted by Dr. Sterner.

She introduced herself, then listened intently as we explained to her that we were determined to beat Kathy's "unbeatable" disease through detoxification, diet and supplements; that we were using no pharmaceuticals whatsoever; and that in the past weeks, even as her legs were getting weaker, she'd seen improvement in swallowing and had sensed movement and tingling in her tongue. We told her that Kathy had her mercury fillings removed and that we were seeing a massage therapist and a chiropractor. We also told her that Kathy was finding it almost impossible to sleep since her fall in the kitchen a couple of weeks earlier.

Much to our surprise, Dr. Sterner thought that we were taking the right approach. She acknowledged that mainstream medicine offered no hope for individuals with ALS. She commented that while there's no medical cure for the disease, that didn't mean we could fully understand or shouldn't pursue all possibilities that might support the body to achieve some level of healing. She even told us that, just the week before, she'd gone to a seminar about the dangers of dental mercury.

Dr. Sterner seemed especially excited to learn about Kathy's improvements. After listening to our description of Kathy's simultaneous decline and improvement, she said it sound like a wave going through her body; where the wave had already passed, healing was beginning, even as the wave continued to move further down her body causing new problems. It seemed like a very perceptive description of what was taking place.

Kathy glanced over at me as best as she could without lifting her head and gave me a little grin. We just may have found the right doctor.

We explained more about the kitchen fall, the neck and shoulder pain and our increasing concern over Kathy's inability to sleep. We told her that we were looking for a local doctor who could help with approving home health care.

We mentioned the recent bladder control incident. Then we asked if she could set Kathy up with intravenous vitamin C.

That's when the wheels came off the cart.

Dr. Sterner said that if she prescribed intravenous vitamin C she'd risk losing her job. She didn't think that it would do any harm and it may even be helpful, but she wasn't in a position to assist us with that without jeopardizing her license, which did not cover her doing such therapies outside the scope of recognized standards of care.

She checked her watch. She'd already gone 10 minutes over the 20 minutes that she was allotted for first appointments and politely told us we'd need to schedule another appointment to discuss what to do about Kathy's sleeping problem and bladder control. As far as the neck pain, she said that she would set us up with a physical therapist, to start right away.

We had hoped for more. But at least getting the physical therapy sessions started would be a step in the right direction.

The woman at the desk scheduled an appointment for Kathy with Dr. Sterner the following Wednesday. Then she called the physical therapy department, explained our situation and got put on hold. Then her call was transferred. Then she got put on hold again. Kathy's head was dropping lower and lower. Her eyes were barely able to stay open.

Finally the receptionist asked for my phone number, put down the phone and explained that the regular physical therapists thought that because of Kathy's ALS she should be seen by a physical therapist from the neurology department. But the neurology department, apparently, couldn't decide when or if they wanted to schedule her, either. So instead of leaving with an appointment to see a physical therapist, as requested by the doctor, we were told that someone would call us later in the day to schedule our sessions.

They never did.

Our goal had been to find a local doctor sympathetic to our cause. That looked promising. But we also hoped to get some immediate help with Kathy's sleeping and pain problems. Those matters had been set aside until another time. The vitamin C drip had been blown off entirely. We left the hospital disappointed.

Once again we were let down by the medical establishment. Kathy would be back at Luther Hospital in a week, but not to see Dr. Sterner.

"Dr. Sterner is too good for this place," I said as I helped Kathy out of the wheelchair and into the car. Kathy nodded in agreement.

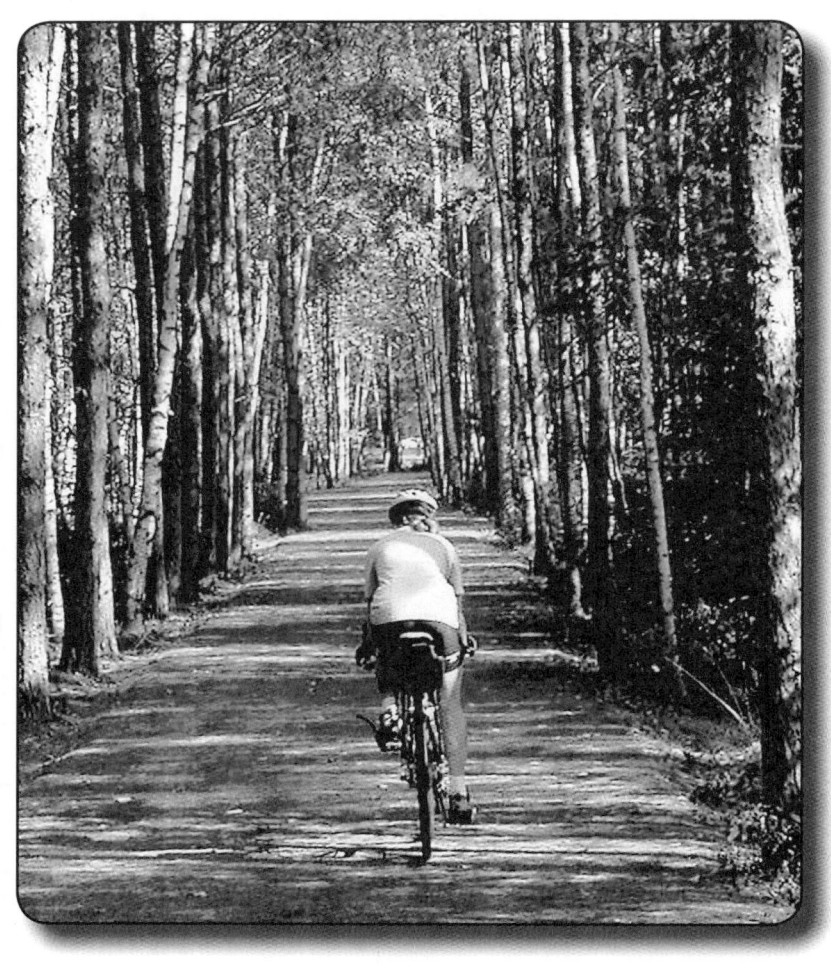

CHAPTER SEVENTEEN
How it All Began

The onset of Kathy's illness began in December 2004 when she first began to notice something wrong with her voice; it started to occasionally change in pitch, like a teenage boy going through puberty.

I didn't notice the change in her voice until about a month later. When I asked about it, she said that it felt like her tongue was swollen and seemed to be coated.

She asked me to look at her tongue to see what I thought. It definitely looked like it had a whitish coating of some sort. She tried to wash it off with her tooth brush. No luck.

The feeling of her tongue being swollen was puzzling. Even though she said it felt like it had gotten larger, that was not at all obvious by looking at it. It looked like a normal tongue with a whitish coating.

In all likelihood, Kathy's dilemma began years earlier when she developed a small, persistent cough. It wasn't a big deal, more like a little hiccup or, as one of the kids described it later, it sounded like she had a little laugh. Small as the cough was, Kathy found it to be quite annoying because it was always there.

Like any person concerned about her health, she made an appointment to see her local medical practitioner, who promptly decided that she—like millions of other folks at the time—had acid reflux disease, also known as gastroesophageal reflux disease or GERD. The solution: one of the funny-named drugs advertised during the nightly news.

Those drugs work by lowering the acidity of stomach secretions. The downside is that your stomach needs those acids to properly digest your food. Too little acid and you don't get all of the nutrients from what you eat.

The GERD medicine did nothing to stop Kathy's cough, but the doctor kept her on it. Eventually, she was switched over to a different brand of the same thing.

Kathy was on this medication for 10 years. We learned much later that it's supposed to be for short-term use only, about two weeks. Then you're supposed to wait at least four months before taking it again.

Kathy had another concern back then. Her face had a red rash, primarily on her cheeks. She was diagnosed with rosacea and prescribed an oral antibiotic and a topical gel to rub onto her face each night before going to bed.

The rosacea didn't go away, but Kathy was advised to keep using both the antibiotic and the gel. She used them for years. Of course, taking antibiotics regularly over time makes them pretty useless and can actually compromise your body's ability to ward off disease. Unfortunately, Kathy trusted her medical provider. She believed that when doctors take an oath to do no harm, they mean it.

Only recently did I discover that the active ingredient in the gel can cause gastric track problems, which Kathy was trying to solve at the time with the GERD medication. I also discovered it can cause problems with the functioning of the nerves outside the spinal cord, numbness, weakness and loss of reflexes; all problems that she would develop.

In March of 2005, we embarked on a week-long bike trip across the state of Missouri. It was cold and damp and on the second morning Kathy work up with gut-wrenching flu. It came on so suddenly that we would have suspected food poisoning had I not eaten the very same food the night before. Aside from her annoying little cough, Kathy was seldom sick, so her sudden illness was a surprise to both of us.

Especially the severity with which it hit her.

Because our car was 200 miles away in St. Charles, we had no choice but to keep going, bicycling more than 50 miles each of the next two days toward our destination.

For a day or two she seemed like she was doing better, pedaling along at about 10 miles per hour. That wasn't nearly as fast as she usually rode, but I was impressed that she was riding at all. Then, on our fourth day, she simply couldn't go on. It took every bit of cheer leading I could muster to keep her going. We ended up walking the last mile into town, arriving just before dark.

The following day we gave a local woman $20 to let us throw our bikes in the back of her pick-up when she went shopping in the next town. We then only had to ride about 10 miles until our next stop, but it took every bit of energy that Kathy had left.

Very early the next morning, I reluctantly left her behind at a bed and breakfast and rode the distance that was planned for two days in one so I could get to the car and come back for her.

When we got back home she decided to go to the clinic again. She told them about her tongue and speech concerns, as well as about her illness on the bike trail. They decided that Kathy had a sinus infection and put her on oral antibiotics, which were in addition to the antibiotics she was already putting on her face.

Kathy's voice continued changing and she began noticeably slurring her words. The coating on her tongue also continued to get worse. She stopped calling it a coating and began to describe the substance on her tongue as "goop."

A few weeks later she went back to the clinic, where they decided that her malady was the result of her long-running acid reflux problem and prescribed an additional dose of the GERD medication.

My sister, who works at a residential health care facility, told Kathy that the coating on her tongue sounded like something called thrush. Kathy did a little research and learned that thrush is a yeast infection that lives in your mouth. Usually your body keeps it under control naturally, but sometimes the fungus can grow uncontrollably on your tongue, especially if your resistance to it is low *because you've been taking antibiotics.*

That sounded like a much more likely cause of the problem than a sinus infection or acid reflux, so, excited to have this new information, Kathy headed back to the doctor, who promptly told her that she was wrong and sent her away.

By this point, Kathy was getting pretty concerned. Her speech kept getting worse, her tongue was getting bumpy as well as coated, and she was beginning to have problems swallowing. Still, no one seemed to take her problem seriously. They had decided it was acid reflux and seemed determined to stick with that diagnosis.

Kathy decided that it was time to see a different doctor, a specialist.

Once again she headed back to her doctor, this time to request a referral to see an eye, nose and throat specialist.

"How did it go?" I asked when she got home.

"Not too well," she said. "I didn't get the referral until I broke down crying." Breaking down crying was not part of Kathy's usual repertoire.

At the end of May 2005, Kathy saw the ENT specialist, who agreed that her slurring and swallowing problems were something to be concerned about. He conducted some swallowing tests and made an appointment for her with a neurologist.

Through all of this, I was simply sitting on the sidelines. After each appointment, she gave me the increasingly frustrating blow-by-blow report.

That changed in the summer of 2005, when she asked that I start going along with her to see the neurologist. She was beginning to sense that something may be seriously wrong and wanted me there to help ask questions and take notes. And ask, we did. We no longer blindly trusted that the first thing a doctor told us was the right thing to do.

Dr. Michael Murphy, the neurologist, was a little leprechaun of a man. From day one, Kathy took a liking to him, in part because he took Kathy seriously, in part because he was a genuinely nice person. Our biggest frustration was that he was always running late and was seldom ready to see us at Kathy's appointed time. After noticing that we were spending far too much time in his waiting room, his nurse, Sandy, suggested that before we left the house, we should give her a call to see how far behind he was. Then, about 30 minutes later, we'd do the same thing. Eventually we'd bike over to his office and get to see him without having to wait very long.

Once we were in his examination room, Dr. Murphy was all ours. He asked a million questions, answered just about as many, and over the course of the summer conducted every test he knew and a few others he'd only read about.

Finally, he said that he had ruled out everything but an uncommon illness called myasthenia gravis.

"At least I'm quite sure that you don't have ALS," he told us.

Myasthenia gravis? ALS? We didn't know much about either one. But obviously, the one that we needed to get acquainted with was myasthenia gravis.

We both started reading up on the disease and Kathy's symptoms did seem to point in that direction. The problems that Kathy had were the problems one should expect with MG, with one big exception: a person with MG may be fine first thing in the morning, but as the day goes on it gets harder to move your muscles. The more you try to move, the more difficult it becomes. With Kathy, there was no difference from one time of day to the next and she usually felt better after doing something physical, such as riding her bike. That summer she rode her bike more than 3,000 miles.

Murphy started Kathy on a drug called prostigmin and told

her to expect to see improvements very quickly.

Nothing changed. No improvement whatsoever.

Instead, it kept getting harder for her to swallow, her speech continued to become more slurred and her tongue was still a mess.

He tried adding predinisone, a steroid that's usually used to reduce swelling. It also decreases the body's natural ability to fight infection by reducing the effectiveness of the immune system.

The goal of both of these drugs was to keep Kathy's immune system from doing what it was supposed to do naturally, so that the drugs could take over and solve her problem artificially. Weakening Kathy's immune system, however, meant that her body couldn't fight off infections and remove toxins on its own.

The predinisone didn't work, either. Because it can be dangerous, Murphy stopped it after a couple of weeks. The prostigmin was continued, even though it had no positive effect. Kathy kept taking it on the assumption that things might be worse without it.

While all of this was going on, the rest of Kathy's life was progressing quite normally. In the spring of 2005 she accepted a half-time job as assistant director at Beaver Creek Reserve, a nearby nature center. It was the perfect job for her, and since it was half time she was able to continue with her garden tending business.

In the summer, she would get up early and head out to the bike trail for a 20- to 30-mile ride before breakfast. Then she would spend the day at either the nature reserve or garden tending. In the evenings, she'd work in her own gardens. Sometimes we'd take the canoe out and enjoy the scenery along one of the nearby rivers. Unless she had to speak with someone, her physical situation didn't cause much of a problem in her daily endeavors. At least not at first.

A major part of Kathy's job at the reserve was to recruit people to present programs and to contact local businesses and individuals about financial support. She loved doing that but most of her contacts needed to be made by phone.

When the people she was calling had to keep asking her to repeat herself, Kathy knew that her days in that job were numbered. By October of 2005, when the people on the other end of the phone could barely understand what she was trying to ask them, she sadly turned in her resignation.

For my part, I could still understand her pretty well, especially at home, when it was quiet and I could see her face. That didn't work on the phone or in social settings.

We were invited to a retirement party for a former co-worker of mine at the Chippewa Valley Museum, where I used to work. Kathy had helped build and design some of the exhibits there as a volunteer, and knew the woman who was retiring. Before we left for the party, Kathy told me that because swallowing had gotten so difficult she wasn't going to even try to eat anything in front of the other people, so we planned to eat supper when we returned.

What we hadn't planned on was how poorly Kathy's voice would carry in a social setting, with many conversations going on at the same time. Try as she might, few people could understand what she said. She had been keeping her health problems to herself, so almost no one knew why she couldn't talk. After a while, when people started up a conversation with her, I would jump in so she wouldn't have to keep straining her voice, trying to be heard and understood. We were the first guests to leave the party. It was the last social event that we agreed to attend.

By this time Kathy was also having strange movements, called fasciculations, in her upper arms. Try to recall a time when you've had a muscle twitch, where one tiny spot in a muscle just kind of jumps or moves on its own. A bit annoying, but no big deal.

Now imagine the same thing, except there are 50 twitches all happening at the same time and it doesn't stop. That's what was going on in Kathy's upper arms.

At night, as we fell asleep holding hands, my arm often rested against hers and sometimes all of the small movements against my skin were more than I could handle; I had to move my arm away from hers.

There was nothing that she could do to stop it. She said that it felt very weird from the inside, too, like worms crawling under her skin. She told me that she was beginning to have similar fasciculations on her tongue. When I looked inside her mouth the sight was very strange indeed; when she tried to stick out her tongue, it took on the appearance of a rapids in a river, with a constant boiling motion.

Dr. Murphy increased the dose of her medicine to stop the fasciculations and it made them even worse. The drug that was supposed to help, had the opposite effect. Within a short time the fasciculations were beginning in her thighs.

By January 2006, Kathy and I were convinced that the diagnosis of myasthenia gravis was wrong and spent most of our winter break researching other illnesses with similar symptoms. We were amazed at how many there were, each with its own name and, individually, considered to be quite unusual.

We thought for sure that we'd figured it out when we discovered something called Kennedy's disease, described by the Kennedy's Disease Association as follows:

> Kennedy's Disease (also known as Spinal Bulbar Muscular Atrophy, SBMA, or Kennedy's Syndrome) is a rare and currently incurable and non-treatable X-linked recessive genetic progressive neuromuscular disease. Both the spinal and bulbar neurons are affected causing muscle weakness and wasting (atrophy) throughout the body which is most noticeable in the extremities (legs/arms), it is especially noticeable in the face and throat, and causes speech and swallowing difficulties, major muscle cramps as well as other symptoms. ... It is estimated that 1 in 40,000 individuals worldwide have Kennedy's Disease. However, many

120

go misdiagnosed or not diagnosed for years.

That didn't sound particularly good, but it did seem like a likely match. We went back to see Dr. Murphy and asked him to take a look at each of the possibilities that we'd found, especially Kennedy's disease. He said that he'd do some more research and tell us what he learned.

One by one, he found a reason why it couldn't be this disease or that disease. He ruled out Kennedy's because it is transmitted genetically and usually only affects males; females are the carriers. None of the males in Kathy's large, extended family had ever exhibited any traits of this disease, so it was very unlikely that's what she had.

By the spring of 2006 we were still stumped. Dr. Murphy finally concurred that it must not be myasthenia gravis because the medicine for it hadn't had any positive effect. Kathy stopped taking the prostigmin and noticed changes within a week.

The most obvious change was in the frequency and severity of the fasciculations in her arms and legs. She still had the twitches, but after she stopped taking the medicine they were not nearly as often and not nearly as severe.

Her voice also improved. It was still mushy, but it was stronger. She had been jotting down specific words to avoid using because they were difficult for her to say. Now she brought out that list and we practiced them together when we went for walks.

The family of eagles in the tree near our home must have been amused listening to our odd conversation as we walked beneath them. I'd say a word, then Kathy would try to repeat it:

Specialize. *Specialize.*

Water drops. *Water drops.*

Something. *Something.*

Church. *Church.*

Poster frame. *Poster frame.*

The holy grail for Kathy was the word *portfolio.* She was

convinced that if she could master that word, she'd be on her way to recovery.

One night, I woke up to her sitting in bed attempting to say portfolio, over and over. She had a dream that she could talk clearly and wanted to see if was real. It didn't sound great, but I could tell that portfolio was the word she was trying to say.

In April of 2006 we decided that we needed a break from all of this medical stuff, so we packed up and headed off to Arkansas. We spent a wonderful week crossing the state, hiking and climbing in a number of its fantastic state parks.

At the end of the week, we went in search of the ivory-billed woodpecker in the Cache River wildlife refuge. We spent eight hours paddling in the bayou that day, chattering away like we hadn't done for a long time. I don't know why she could talk so well that day. She didn't either. Perhaps it was the incredible silence that shrouded us among the Cyprus and tupelo trees. Maybe it was the high humidity. Maybe the adrenalin of being on an adventure.

Whatever the reason, it was wonderful. When we got back to the little ma and pa motel, Sam and Mary, the older couple who owned it, invited us to their living quarters to hear all about our day's journey. Kathy wasn't sure if she wanted to go, since she didn't expect she'd be able to participate in the conversation. We agreed that I'd do most of the talking and we would stay for only a few minutes.

An hour and a half later we finally went back to our room. Kathy had been able to participate in the conversation quite well; they only asked her to repeat herself a couple of times. That night we went to bed tired and happy. We slept great, which was a milestone in itself.

I'll never forget that day, not only because of the wonderful time paddling through the swamp, but because it was the last extended conversation that I or anyone else ever had with Kathy.

After that, her voice kept going downhill.

CHAPTER EIGHTEEN
ex • pert (ek'spert) *n.* synonym for hopeless

In May of 2006 we went to the neurology clinic at the University of Wisconsin hospital in Madison to try to get a better sense of what was going on. We had appointments scheduled with a swallowing specialist and a neurologist. Dr. Murphy said he had pulled a few strings to get them to see us.

The first person we saw was the swallowing specialist. Dr. Murphy wanted us to see her because she could conduct a test in Madison that he was unable to have done locally.

We sat in a room and the swallowing doctor pretty much just talked with us and made Kathy do her best to talk back. By this time, Kathy had begun using a white board quite often to communicate, but the specialist wanted to hear Kathy's voice. After about half an hour, the doctor announced that she was done.

"What about the swallowing test?" Kathy asked? We'd come a long ways to see a specialist to not do the test.

The specialist told us that there was no need to do the tests; she'd learned enough just by listening to Kathy talk to be sure that it wasn't myasthenia gravis. If it was MG, she explained, Kathy's voice would have dropped off to almost nothing during the half hour she'd been talking.

We had already concluded on our own that it wasn't myasthenia gravis. We were in Madison because we wanted to hear from someone who knew more than we did.

We asked her what else she thought it might be and for suggestions about what could be done to help. She told us that we could talk about that further with the neurologist and walked us to the neurology clinic.

After a long wait, we were taken to an examination room and visited by not one, but three doctors, all wearing white coats. Actually, they weren't all doctors: One was the neurologist, the second was a resident and the third was a medical student. Each spoke with a different accent.

The neurologist began his examination. He had Kathy lie on a table and he twisted and bent her legs, calling out numbers as he did this to his white-coated partners. Then he had Kathy lift her arms up and down and checked their range of motion. He pushed against her forehead to check the strength of her neck and continued to call out numbers to the other two.

Continuing the drill, most of which we'd already seen a dozen times in Eau Claire, he asked Kathy to stick out her tongue and then move it sideways to touch the inside of her cheeks. She couldn't stick it out beyond her teeth and had no side-to-side movement at all. Then Dr. Whitecoat ran a small stick under the arches of her feet, from heel to toe, as if he was tickling her, and watched to see which way her toes moved.

During all of this he kept a running monologue with the other two white coats, one of who was taking notes. None of what he said made any sense to Kathy or me. It was all numbers and medical jargon.

When he was done poking and prodding, Kathy asked him what could be done to improve her voice and swallowing.

"You have a very serious illness," was all he told her. But, he said, we were in luck because one of his colleagues was an internationally known expert in the area of her disease, and he would talk to the expert and get him to see us. Then he wrote out a prescription and handed it to Kathy.

"I know my colleague will want you on this medication," he said. "Get this filled on the way home and start it tonight. Don't wait until tomorrow."

After he politely exited the room, Whitecoat Number Two, the resident, did a few other tests, explaining to the student, not to us, what he was doing. Then he told us that we could leave.

We were supposed to tell Dr. Murphy what we'd learned when we got back to Eau Claire, but we didn't really have any idea what to tell him. So before we left the examination room, Kathy asked the resident if he could tell us what it was they decided that she had.

"Bulbar neuromuscular disease," he said. "Sometimes it's called neuromuscular disease with bulbar presentation."

Kathy asked him to write it down so we'd be sure what he said. Then we took his note and the prescription and left.

We weren't quite sure what to make of our visit to the big leagues. We were both disappointed and optimistic.

Disappointed because the anticipated swallowing test didn't happen and because no one had offered any concrete suggestions to help.

Optimistic because Kathy was being put on a new medication that must be pretty powerful or they wouldn't have stressed that we start it immediately. We were also happy that we would soon be seeing one of the top docs in the world for Kathy's disease, whatever it was.

After heading in the wrong direction for nearly a year, with the misdiagnosis of myasthenia gravis, we thought that maybe we were finally on the right track.

It was late by the time we got back to Eau Claire from Madison. Before going home, we stopped at the nearest Walgreens. They didn't stock the prescribed medicine and sent us to another Walgreens, on the opposite side of town. Since Dr. Whitecoat had stressed that we start the drug immediately, we drove across town to get it.

Kathy waited in the car while I went in to have the prescription filled. As the pharmacist handed me a little white bag with a label stapled to the top, he said, "I'm so sorry for you. ALS is an awful disease. You will be in my prayers."

Sorry? ALS? Prayers?

I asked him to explain. He told me that the drug, Rilutek, was prescribed for only one disease—ALS. He said that when he was in pharmacy school, not long ago, he'd been following its development and research.

"A very expensive drug," he said. "It's a good thing that your insurance covers it." As I left, he again gave me his condolences and said that we'd be in his prayers.

When we got home, I told Kathy what he said about the drug being for ALS. I didn't mention the condolences or prayers.

After all of the experts Kathy had seen, she learned that she had been diagnosed with ALS from *me*, after I'd been told by a pharmacist at Walgreens.

Since we had been led to believe that Kathy did not have ALS, we never took the time to learn anything about it. Immediately, Kathy and I started googling "ALS" and "bulbar motor neuron disease." It turns out that motor neuron disease is what ALS is called in other parts of the world. Maybe the three doctors, none of who seemed to be from the United States, thought they had told us what she had, but communication only works when everyone uses the same words.

The "bulbar" part of the name indicated that the disease first presented itself in the throat and tongue, which meant it would first cause difficulty in speaking and swallowing. About 90 percent of the time, ALS begins with weakness in the legs and arms and ends with the inability to speak or swallow. Leave it to Kathy to do things differently than most everyone else.

Almost every description of ALS that we found included the same three words. Over and over we read "incurable" and "always fatal," usually within three to five years.

We were glad that soon we would be seeing a world-renown expert in ALS and we appreciated that Dr. Whitecoat had gotten us started right away on the one medicine approved for ALS.

Two weeks later we headed back to Madison, confident that if anybody could help Kathy, it would be Dr. Renown. He only accepted one or two new patients a week and only on Mondays, so we were glad to be able to get in.

He really was world-renown. We googled his name and discovered that several years earlier he'd convened an international panel to draft uniform standards for diagnosing ALS. He was also lead researcher for a different and promising drug.

Before we met with Dr. Renown, an associate conducted a number of tests to confirm Dr. Whitecoat's suspicions. Because of Kathy's trouble communicating, she asked that I stay with her during her tests. I was able to understand much of what she said, but a stranger usually couldn't. I think that she also felt reassured having me at her side, although I doubt that I was very reassuring during these tests.

I hate getting shots. I don't even like mosquito bites and can vividly recall how much it hurts when a hypodermic needle pokes into a muscle. It still makes me cringe.

For one of Kathy's tests, the doctor pushed a long, thick, needle-type probe into her back, arm and leg, specifically aiming for muscle. Once the probe was in the muscle he wiggled it around while monitoring the electrical impulses being sent through her nerves. He did this over and over and over in different muscles, on different parts of her body.

Kathy never complained once. I wanted to jump up and shout, "stop it, you're torturing her." But I followed her lead and sat quietly, gritting my teeth. There's no way that I could have handled those tests.

Following a long wait, which by then we'd come to expect from neurologists, we finally got to meet Dr. Renown, a gruff, overweight fellow who looked as if he'd be unable to walk up a flight of stairs without puffing and panting.

He asked the same questions and did some of the same movement tests that everyone else had done. Then he came up with something new. He had Kathy go out in the hallway and run between a couple of lines taped to the floor while he timed her with a stopwatch. She did great. She liked that sort of test.

Then he had her sit down, put her right hand on her right knee and flip it over, from palm up to palm down, as many times as she could in 30 seconds. The number of flips was dutifully recorded without comment. Then he did the same thing with her left hand.

After recording the timed results of a few more simple tests, like standing on one leg at a time, he told us that the examinations confirmed what was suspected: Kathy had ALS.

He invited her to participate in a day-long assessment, a month later, with a team of specialists. The assessment team, together, would help develop her treatment plan. That sounded promising.

Dr. Renown wrote out a couple of prescriptions. In addition to renewing the prescription for Rilutek, he wrote out one that he thought may help with Kathy's increasing problem of drooling. He mentioned that it was actually for some other disease, but it had a side effect of causing severe dry mouth.

He also told Kathy to cut back drastically on her exercising. At that time of year, Kathy was bicycling about 20 miles every day. Just two days earlier, she and I had been biking on one of the newest and most beautiful bike trails in northern Wisconsin. The paved trail wound through the north woods, along the shore of Crystal Lake, then back into the forest. It was a wonderful ride that included quite a few short, steep hills.

We had ridden about 25 miles that day and when we finished, Kathy was feeling great. Even though she could barely speak or swallow, she still had excellent strength in her legs. She wasn't the slightest bit winded by the exertion of the hills. Very little made her feel more alive than riding her bicycle in a beautiful setting.

Dr. Renown, who didn't look like he'd ever been on a bike, instructed her to cut back to no more than one short bike ride every four days... and no hills. "If you're used to riding 120 miles a week," he said, "cut it back to 12."

He also instructed her to start adding more fat to her diet because she was losing so much weight. There was no question that losing weight was a problem. She'd been doing her best to maintain her diet, but eating had become very difficult. Because she couldn't move the food around in her mouth with her tongue, it was a challenge to chew. Once she did get her food chewed, it was almost impossible to get it into her throat. And once it was in her throat, it took three or four tries before she could get it to go down. Trying to wash it down with water only made things worse and caused her to choke.

The swallowing specialist in Eau Claire had taken video X-rays of her swallowing and discovered that she had the best chance of the food going down if she lowered her chin and turned her head to the left.

So each bite of food became a multi-step process. First, get the food chewed, which often meant moving it under her teeth with a spoon or with her finger. Once it was chewed she had to toss it back or push it into her throat. And finally, she needed to tip and turn her head to try, usually several times, to get it to go down.

Going through all of this in public was out of the question. When we had company, it wasn't uncommon for her to discretely get up and go into the bathroom to try to maneuver the food into the right position. After everyone was gone, she'd usually eat again, without having to worry about choking or grossing out her fellow diners.

My sister, who works in a long-term health care facility, suggested that Kathy consider a feeding tube. Dr. Renown had also recommended a feeding tube as a way for Kathy to get more nutrition.

At the end of our appointment, he shook our hands, said he'd see us in a month, then instructed us to go to the respiratory clinic where they would conduct some more tests.

We weren't sure why. Kathy didn't have any problems breathing. Besides that, they had already diagnosed her, so what were they hoping to learn?

Turned out it didn't matter. After making us wait for almost an hour, the respiratory staff wasn't able to conduct the tests because Kathy couldn't close her lips tightly enough around the testing apparatus.

I wasn't a witness to what happened—they made me sit in the hall, saying there wasn't enough room for me where they did the tests—but when Kathy came out, she was very sad. She said they scolded her for wasting their time.

A month later, we were back. We weren't looking forward to the drive and the required night's lodging, but we were looking forward to the team assessment, which would lead to Kathy's treatment plan.

Once again, we had to sit for more than an hour in the waiting room. After we got into the examination room, though, it was a non-stop marathon of experts.

In the course of six hours, Kathy and I met with eight different specialists. We stayed in the same room while they rotated through, with few breaks.

A speech therapist and her assistant concluded that Kathy was having difficulty speaking.

Duh.

They told Kathy that maybe she could try using a white board and write her messages. She'd already been doing that for several months.

They gave us some promotional literature about machines that could help her communicate. She could type her message onto a keyboard and it would speak the words aloud. We'd heard about them and Kathy was an excellent typist, so it sounded like a good idea. We asked if they could dem-

130

onstrate it for us.

They could, but they'd have to see if they could find a machine, first. Eventually, about four hours later, the assistant showed up with a little speaking machine that reminded me of something you might find at Toys 'R' Us. He explained that it was quite old and out-of-date and was, in fact, no longer actually being used. Kathy managed to talk him into letting her take it home so that she could try it out for a couple of weeks.

The speech therapist also showed Kathy some charts that included pictures of things like a glass of water, a plate of food, a toilet and a bed. She explained that Kathy would use something like this, connected to a head pointer, to make people aware of her needs when she could no longer communicate in any other way.

Another expert, a physical therapist, felt up Kathy's arms and shoulders and declared that her muscles were already beginning to atrophy, so we should begin to plan for the day when she could no longer move at all. I was given information about how to widen the doors in our home so that her wheel chair would fit through them. They also gave me suggestions for remodeling the bathroom and building a ramp to the back door.

A respiratory therapist brought in something called a cough machine. This was for situations when Kathy was choking and unable to get the phlegm out of her throat. The therapist tried to demonstrate it for us, but couldn't get it to work. Finally, after fumbling with it for 10 or 15 minutes, she simply *told* us what it should be doing. It was reassuring to know that, in an emergency, I could *tell* Kathy what the machine was *supposed* to be doing to keep her from choking to death.

A representative of the Muscular Dystrophy Association, which funded some of Dr. Renown's research, came in to tell us about the many wonderful things they could do to help, including assistance with paying for things like the cough machine.

Because we were out of the rep's service area, she wrote down Kathy's name, address and phone number and told us that we should expect a call from an MDA person closer to our home, and that person would explain how we'd go about applying for funds and other benefits.

We never did receive a call from them. But in a month or two we started getting their newsletter, bragging about all the organization's many achievements, along with a request for a donation.

Another expert came in to talk with us about Social Security and Medicare. She explained how lucky we were: because Kathy had ALS she'd get fast-tracked into the system and wouldn't have to wait the usual period for benefits to kick in.

Lucky? What we heard was, if you have ALS you'll die so quickly that if you don't get your benefits right away, you won't have time to get them at all.

The last person we saw was Dr. Renown. He grabbed his stop watch and ran Kathy through the same timed drills as before. She ran up and down the hallway. She flipped her hands over on her knees. She stood on one leg.

We asked him what sort of progress Kathy could anticipate. We meant progress of healing, but he looked at it differently.

"Our goal is to slow the progression of the disease enough so that we can discover a cure," he said. In other words, Kathy should expect to keep getting worse while *they* tried to discover a cure. It was all up to them. Kathy was simply along for the ride.

Finally, Kathy asked him, flat out, in pretty clear speech: "Will I die?"

"Everyone who has ALS will eventually die," he said.

Then he told us that the members of the assessment team with whom we had spent the day, would get together to decide the best plan for Kathy. He said we would get their recommendations in the mail.

As promised, about a week later we received an envelope from the ALS clinic. There was only one thing inside. A hand-written prescription for LifeLine, the alert service that lets you summon an ambulance by pushing a button hung around your neck.

A button wasn't the only thing they'd hung around Kathy's neck. They'd given her a death sentence with no possibility of pardon.

A month later, in August, Kathy was supposed to see Dr. Renown again. She was even practicing her hand flips so she could show him that she was improving, not getting worse.

The day before we were to drive back to Madison, we looked at each other and knew what we were thinking.

"Should we go?" Kathy asked, using the speech synthesizer we'd rigged up on our own.

"Why bother," I said. "They have nothing to offer."

"I agree," she typed. She smiled as best as she could, then quickly started hitting the keys. "Call him up and cancel our appointment. Tell him he won't get to keep timing my demise."

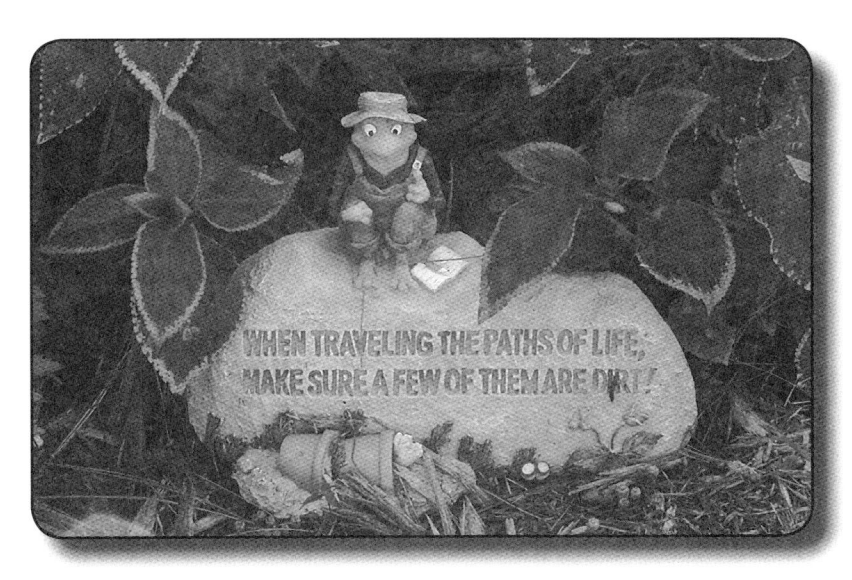

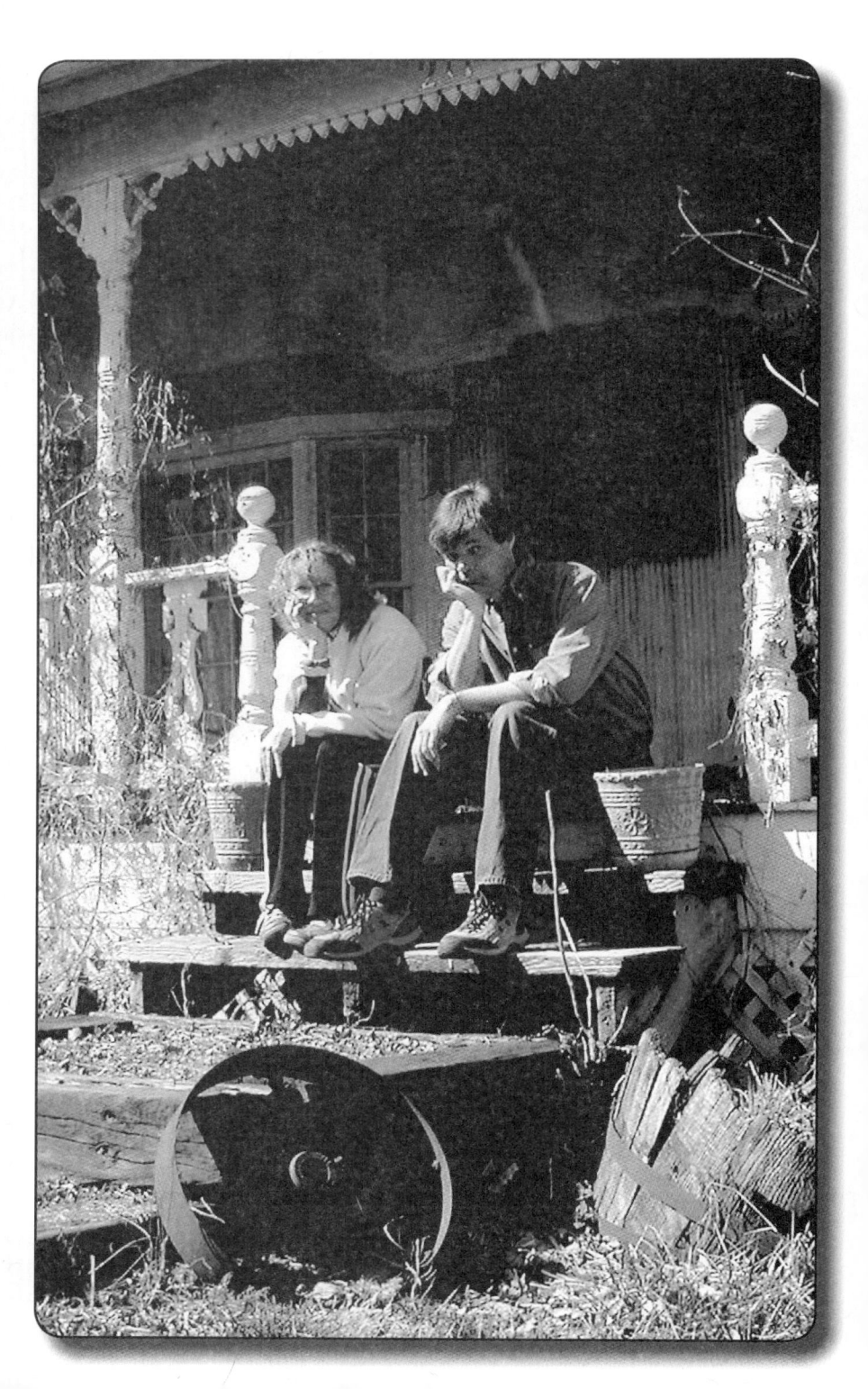

CHAPTER NINETEEN
The Feeding Tube Fiasco

Near the end of June 2006, Kathy met with a local gastroenterologist to discuss putting in the feeding tube. Upon seeing how little ability she had to swallow and how much weight she was losing, he worked her into his schedule the same week.

The type of device that Kathy had placed is called a PEG tube, which stands for percutaneous endoscopic gastrostomy tube. We usually just called it a feeding tube.

The feeding tube is placed directly into the stomach through the abdominal wall and sticks out of your belly, kind of like an umbilical cord. In some ways, that's a pretty good description because the feeding tube, like an umbilical cord, becomes your conduit for nutrition.

The part of the tube that's inside the stomach has an enlargement, similar to the cap of a mushroom, so that it can't easily be pulled out.

Kathy had been researching feeding tubes for a couple of weeks and went from knowing nothing about them to being quite well informed. Like so many of the things she researched, some of the information seemed contradictory. Much of what she read about feeding tubes seemed biased in favor of the companies that profit from associated products, such as pumps, bags and formula.

Most of the information she found explained that the tube

was very narrow and that commercial formula was required in order to keep it from clogging. Commercial formula was the correct thickness and included something to keep it from leaving a residue. Noncommercial formulas and normal food were not recommended because they would clog up the narrow tubing.

Doing some further research, however, Kathy discovered that feeding tubes come in different sizes. On a blog, written by a person who had a PEG tube, she learned that one can request a larger than normal tube that isn't as likely to clog and, even better, allows the user to blend up her own food and not have to rely on the canned formula.

That seemed like a good idea, especially since Kathy was already trying to eat mostly organic and locally grown foods and wanted to continue with her healthy diet.

The standard tube isn't much bigger around than the insert in a ballpoint pen. The tube Kathy wanted was about the size of a crayon.

Even though it wasn't the doctor's standard practice, and he didn't quite seem to understand why Kathy would want to go through all of the work of blending her own food, he agreed to put in the larger size tube. Kathy could be quite convincing.

The doctor told Kathy that the surgery was very simple and could be done on an outpatient basis at the hospital. That seemed like good news, although my sister had warned us that they'd try to send us home too soon. She had seen cases where the patient was released too early and had to return to the hospital.

Kathy couldn't eat anything the night before the surgery and was given something to clean out her digestive track. That was no surprise. She was also informed by someone from the hospital that she would need to drink some barium-containing liquid six to eight hours before the surgery. This would allow a radiologist to X-ray her belly and see exactly where her stomach was located, so that the surgeon would know the correct spot to make his incision.

Kathy had to swallow the same liquid barium a couple of times earlier at that hospital when they conducted her swallowing tests. She said she could barely get it down then, not because of the taste or consistency, but because she couldn't swallow and it caused her to choke. Several months had passed and her swallowing abilities had gotten worse. She didn't think that she could swallow it safely.

Nonetheless, they said that it needed to be done and told me to come to the lab and pick it up.

The afternoon before her surgery, I biked over to the hospital to pick up the barium. I was directed to the lab, where I informed them I was there to pick up the barium for Kathy. At Kathy's request, I reiterated her concern that she wouldn't be able to swallow it.

They told me that she could swallow it if she tried; that it didn't taste that bad; that maybe she could hold her nose when she drank it. They didn't seem to grasp the concept that when I said "she wouldn't be able to swallow it," I meant that literally.

Finally they told me that if she wasn't able to swallow it on her own, then I should bring her to the hospital at four a.m. and they would "pour it down her throat with a tube." That seemed more like a threat than an offer.

I told them that I would take it home with me and see what Kathy thought.

They handed me a paper cup, like a shake cup from McDonalds, two-thirds full of a grayish liquid.

"What am I supposed to do with that?" I asked.

"Take it home and give it to your wife to drink."

"I can't carry that home, I'm on my bicycle."

They looked at me like I was insane.

"Could you put it in a jar, so it won't spill?" I asked.

They spent a good 60 seconds looking, then told me they didn't have any extra jars. Eventually, someone managed to find a plastic lid and snapped that over the cup. I said that I was still concerned about getting it home safely, without spilling it. They told me that I should go back home and get my car; they'd set it behind the counter until I returned.

I decided to take my chances carrying it in one hand.

When I got home, Kathy took one look at it and wrote, "I can't swallow that." She explained that she'd been asked to swallow far smaller amounts for her other tests and couldn't always do it. There was no way that she could swallow all of that without choking.

I told her that her only other option was to get up at 4 a.m. and go to the hospital so they could pour it down her throat with a tube.

She asked me to call the surgeon, to see if he could suggest a way for her to swallow it at home.

He seemed very puzzled by my question. The technique that he was planning to use to locate the incision point in Kathy's stomach didn't involve swallowing barium, or anything else. He knew that Kathy couldn't swallow and that wouldn't work.

Someone at the hospital had apparently assumed on their own that he'd be using the barium method, because that's what was often done. Had Kathy swallowed the barium, she may have had to reschedule her surgery.

The next morning, Kathy was sedated and a flexible scope with a light at the end was fed through her mouth, down her throat and into her stomach. In a darkened room, a spot of light shone through her stomach wall to let the surgeon know precisely where to make a small incision in her belly and stomach.

Then a suture was attached to the scope and, with the suture trailing behind, it was pulled back out of her mouth. Next, the suture was removed from the scope and attached to the feeding tube. By pulling on the end of the suture that was still sticking out of her belly, the surgeon pulled the tube through her mouth and throat, into her stomach and out through the incision. The mushroom shaped bulge at the end of the tube kept it from pulling out of her stomach. Once it was in place, a small stopper was slid over the tube so that everything stayed in place. Pretty nifty, actually. The whole procedure took only about 20 minutes.

When he was finished, the surgeon came out and talked with me in the waiting room and said that the operation had gone smoothly. He expected Kathy could leave in a few hours, once the anesthesia wore off and the nurses were certain she was in stable condition.

He also said something else: Kathy had no trace in her esophagus of ever having had acid reflux disease. Her throat was in perfect condition, without even the slightest bit of scarring from stomach acid. She had been taking the prescribed GERD medication for all those years and hadn't needed it. Besides that, it never helped with her cough. Much later we learned that a small persistent cough is one of the first symptoms of mercury poisoning.

While Kathy and I were in the outpatient recovery room, a nutritionist came in to talk with us about the new diet that Kathy would be on. She brought along a few sample cans of Nutren formula, a couple of gravity bags and some large syringes.

The nutritionist said that she had checked with our insurance company to find out which medical supply company they worked with, and had ordered additional formula, bags and syringes for us, to be delivered directly to our house. She said they'd be there by the time we got home. She also said that she arranged for a home health care nurse to come to our house to teach us how to use the feeding tube.

That seemed like pretty good service. We hadn't thought about how to arrange for those things, and now we didn't have to worry about it.

Kathy asked if there were any special recipes or restrictions we needed to be aware of when blending up our food. The nutritionist pointed out that we wouldn't have to worry about that because Kathy would be exclusively using the canned formula, which included all of the nutrients, vitamins and minerals that she needed. There was no need for anything else.

The nutritionist explained that the formula came in various calorie levels. Kathy would start out with the higher calorie formula five or six times a day, then, once she regained her weight, would change to a formula with fewer calories or reduce the number of feedings. Nothing to it.

Kathy still wanted to know about blending up her own food.

Finally the nutritionist admitted that she didn't know anything about doing that, but that the home health care nurse could probably tell us about it when we met with her at home.

By the time the nutritionist left, Kathy was feeling quite a bit of pain from her surgery. The hospital staff decided to keep her in the recovery room for a few more hours.

After the few more hours were over, Kathy felt even worse and they decided to admit her. By the time she was in her room she was feeling awful.

To relieve her pain, Kathy was given some morphine. That helped the pain, but also did quite a number on her. She became hot and sweaty and as limp as an old dish rag.

She pushed the button on the side of the bed to call a nurse. "Yes, what do you need?" came a voice from a small speaker along the side of the bed.

When Kathy came to the hospital she could barely speak. After the scope and PEG tube were run down her throat, she couldn't so much as make a sound. Kathy couldn't respond, and it didn't immediately occur to me that I should.

No one came.

After a few minutes Kathy tried again. This time when the nurse responded over the speaker I told her that Kathy was feeling very ill after the morphine. I also pointed out that Kathy couldn't speak and they would need to come to the room when she pushed the button. I was planning to go home for the night and wanted to make sure that if Kathy called for help they would respond.

When the nurse did come, Kathy indicated to her that she

needed to go to the bathroom. The nurse said that she could use the bathroom in the room, but Kathy was too dizzy and too weak to walk the few steps to get there on her own. The nurse helped her out of bed, then walked her slowly to the bathroom.

Trusting that she was in good hands, I went back to watching TV. A short while later I heard something fall in the bathroom; it sounded like a plastic water pitcher bouncing off the sink and onto the floor. I didn't think much of it.

After a while I began wondering what could possibly be taking Kathy and the nurse so long in the bathroom. I got up, and just as I was at the bathroom door, the nurse walked in from the hallway.

She quickly opened the bathroom door, and crumpled in the corner, head cocked up against the hard, tile wall, lay Kathy. The nurse had left her in the bathroom alone.

Kathy hadn't been able to call to let anyone know that she was finished, and when no one came for her she tried to get off the toilet on her own, but instead fell into the corner, hitting her head against the wall. That was the sound I heard.

The wayward nurse turned around, stepped back into the room and pulled a cord on the wall. Within moments there were half a dozen people in the room trying to decide what to do. They checked Kathy's head to see if she had any bumps or cuts. They speculated about a possible concussion. They didn't want to move her until they were sure she didn't have any broken bones. All the while I am getting more and more angry.

When they finally decided that it was safe to move her, they put her into a wheelchair and checked a few more things. Then they rolled her back to her bed and helped her get in.

"This won't happen again," the nurse assured me.

"That's for sure," I said. "I am not leaving her side until she gets outta this place. If she has to go to the bathroom,

I'm taking her."

They told me that I was welcome to sleep in the extra bed. I pushed it up next to her so that we could hold hands.

A couple hours later, Kathy let me know that she was again feeling a lot of pain in her belly. I pressed the call button, and when the nurse-in-the-box asked what I wanted, I told her that Kathy was in quite a bit of pain.

The solution? Give her more morphine!

This time the results were even worse. Kathy started sweating and got so limp that she could barely move. Then she started to throw up blood. She could not swallow or spit and did not have the strength to turn her head.

I hit the call button, but there was no time to wait for the nurse. I grabbed the suction tube off the wall behind the bed, tipped Kathy's head to the side and started suctioning the blood out of her mouth and throat.

"Yes, can I help you?" came the little voice inside the speaker.

I'd had all I could take. I ran down the hall as fast as I could to the nursing station and interrupted the chattering nurses with a frantic "Get down here right away. She's throwing up blood, she's choking!"

The nurses were the ones I wanted to choke.

Neither Kathy nor I even tried to get any rest after that. We just wanted to get out of there and get home.

The doctor came by the next morning and released us. I have no idea how much he heard about the fiascoes of the night before, but he surely was nice to us. We had no complaints about him; it was the incompetent nursing care that could have killed Kathy.

A day or two later, someone called from the hospital, I believe it was a nursing supervisor, and asked me how Kathy was doing. The supervisor said that she'd heard there may have been a problem and wanted to make sure that everything was okay. My interpretation of the call was that they were trying to ascertain if we would file a lawsuit. That wasn't something we even considered. We had other things to worry about. We were just glad to be out of that place.

When we got back home, boxes with formula, bags, syringes and a long metal pole were sitting by the back door. A few hours later, the home health care nurse stopped by to teach us how to use the feeding tube.

She showed us how to pour the formula from the can into the plastic gravity bag and hang it from the pole, and how to get the flow of formula started. She demonstrated how to uncap the feeding tube and flush it out with water from the syringe. She instructed us how to connect the tiny hose from the gravity bag to the feeding tube and explained that it should be adjusted to drip from the bag very slowly.

She cautioned us against doing this too fast. It should take at least 45 minutes to an hour to finish one 8.45 ounce can of formula. There was another caution: following her feeding, Kathy was not supposed to lie down for at least 30 minutes. It was best if she just stayed sitting in the chair.

We were supposed to do this five or six times a day, which meant dedicating anywhere between six-and-a-quarter and nine hours a day to feedings.

The home health nurse waited with us during the hour it took for the inaugural can of Nutren to drain into Kathy's stomach. During that time, Kathy asked her to explain how we would go about using our own food. Was there a certain way to blend it? Did some foods work better than others? What should we use to thin it?

The nurse had no idea. She didn't know of anyone who had ever done that. She checked with the other nurses at her office, but none of them had any experience with it either.

She did suggest that if we tried it, we should use the syringe, because blended food probably wouldn't flow through the gravity bag's narrow tube. She also speculated that we would need to do it very slowly, no faster than the 45 to 60 minutes it would take for a can of formula.

When it came right down to it, if we were going to use our

own food, we were on our own.

For the first couple weeks, Kathy existed completely on Nutren and began gaining back her weight. She tried to continue eating some food through her mouth, but that didn't last long. Within a couple of weeks she completely lost her ability to swallow.

Even though she didn't have much energy to do anything else, it wasn't easy for Kathy to sit for an hour while the formula drained into her belly. She was extremely bored. She was terribly sad. "I want my life back," she wrote on her board.

We figured out a couple of places to hang the gravity bag that would be more enjoyable. Her favorite place to read in the summer was sitting in her Adirondak chair in the front garden. I found a wrought iron plant hanger and stuck it in the ground next to the chair. It worked fine for holding the gravity bag and looked less medical than lugging out the shiny metal pole.

In her office, I mounted a decorative plant hanger on the wall next to her desk. That gave her the opportunity, while "eating," to spend time at her computer sending e-mails and researching possible cures for her disease.

After she regained most of her weight, we decided to start adding real food back into her diet. We made a typical meal, with the same foods that we usually ate, then we each filled our plates with the amount of food that we'd normally eat. My food stayed on the plate and hers went into the blender, with extra milk to make it thinner.

It worked pretty well. She sucked the liquefied food into the syringe, then squeezed it into her feeding tube. Instead of stretching the feeding out over an hour, as recommended, she matched the rate at which I was eating. We figured that instead of duplicating the routine for the formula, it made more sense to replicate normal eating patterns. If she could eat an entire meal in 20 minutes by way of her mouth, why should it take three times that long to do it with a tube?

It was almost like old times. We both started and finished

our meals together. That felt good.

Kathy weened herself off the formula over a couple of weeks, first replacing one meal a day, then two, then all of them.

By the end of Summer 2006, about the same time that Kathy said farewell to Dr. Renown, she also ended her relationship Nutren.

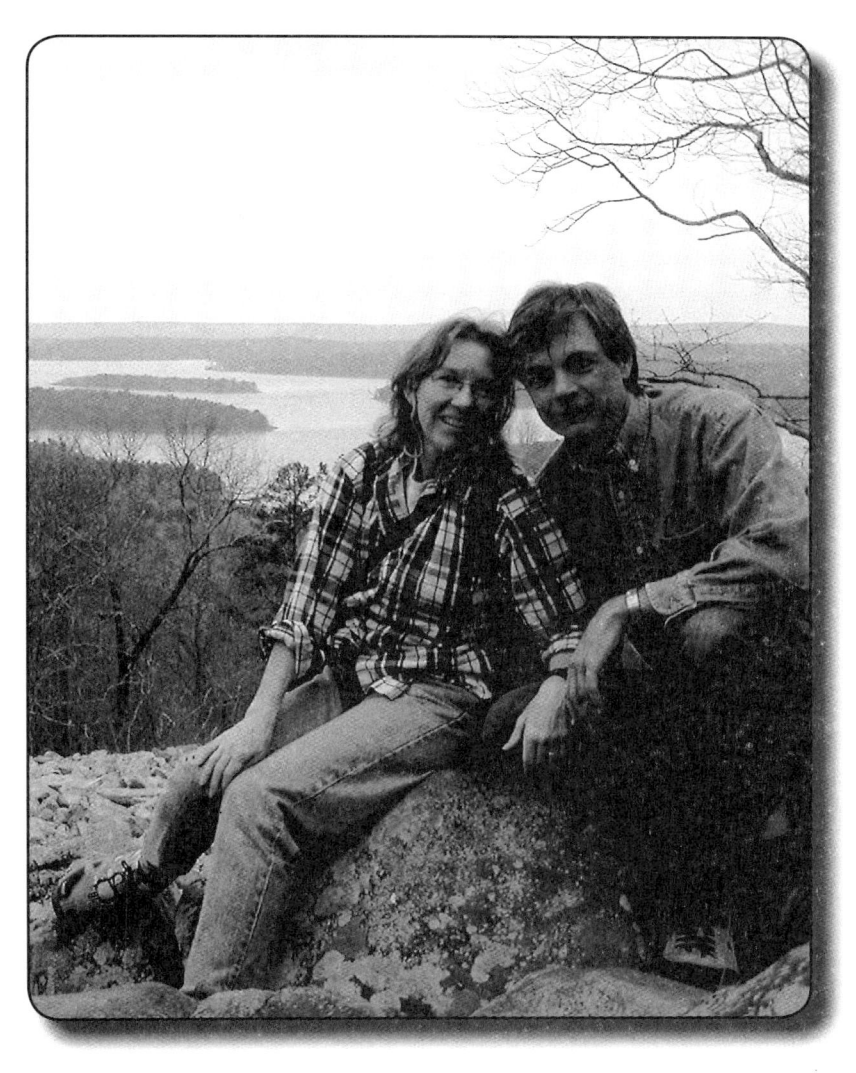

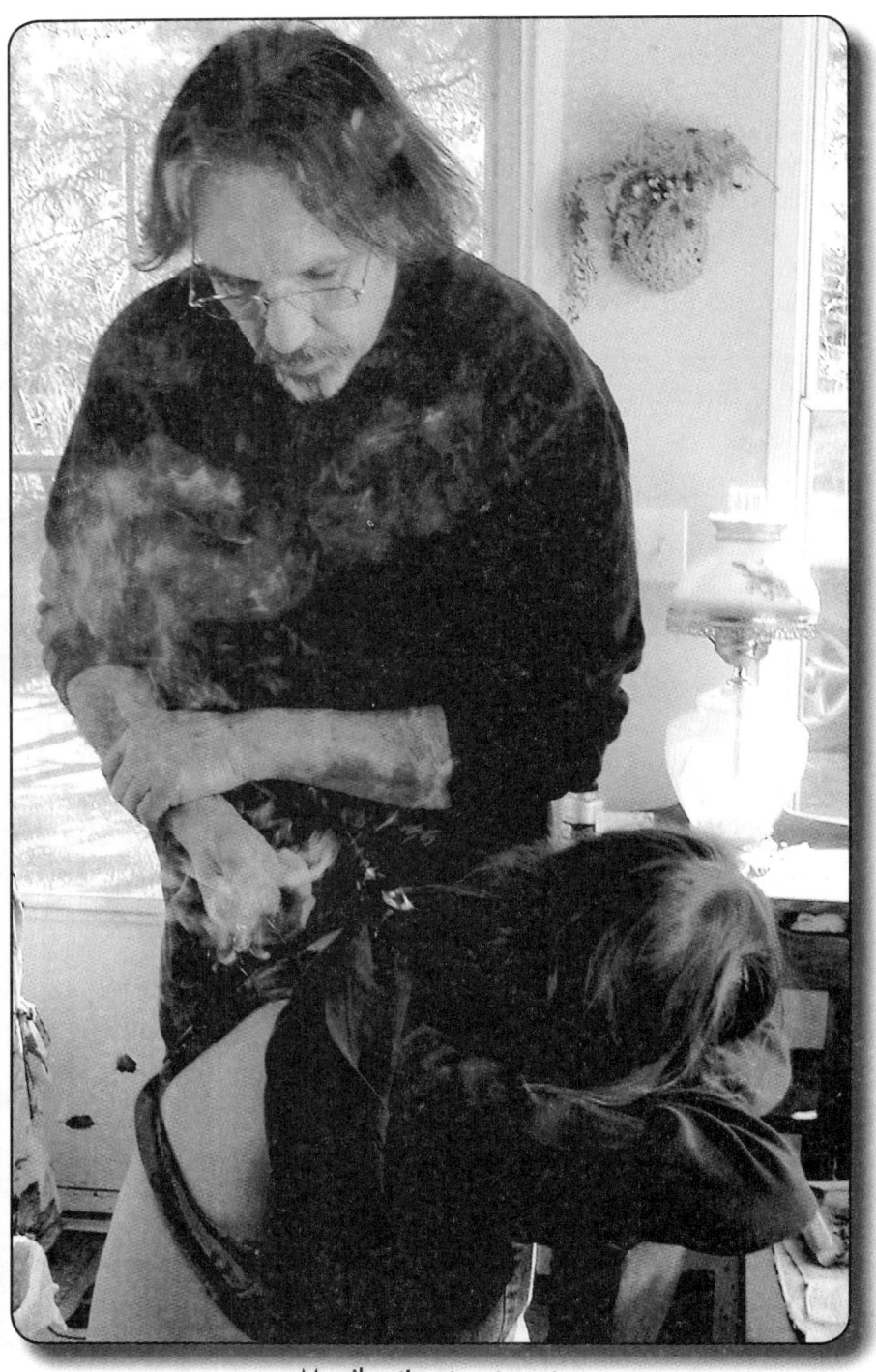

Moxibustion treatment.

CHAPTER TWENTY
An Alternative to What?

Shortly after Kathy decided that her diagnosis of myasthenia gravis was wrong, she began on her own researching and trying treatments outside of established medicine, even as we continued searching for new answers within the field of neurology.

During the next year and a half, Kathy increasingly sought the assistance of health care professionals who practiced alternative medicine. The umbrella terms alternative and complementary medicine mean different things to different people, but for us, alternative meant acupuncture, chiropractic, acupressure, therapeutic massage, herbs, dietary changes, dietary supplements and vitamins. We even did a little experimenting with magnets.

In the early part of 2006, Kathy's brother, a licensed acupuncturist from St. Louis, recommended that she look for someone locally to begin acupuncture treatments. We found a chiropractor in a neighboring town who also did acupuncture, and made an appointment. After listening to Kathy's symptoms, he decided to connect the acupuncture needles to a low-voltage electrical current, in the hope of stimulating her nerves. He placed the needles primarily in her upper chest and neck, trying to work in the areas closest to her problems, which at the time were limited to swallowing and speaking. We discussed the possibility of placing needles in her tongue, but decided against that.

He told us that we should not expect to see much change immediately and recommended a minimum of 10 sessions. After six visits, Kathy decided to stop. She didn't notice any improvement and the 50-mile drive and $100 fee each visit kept her from continuing. He may well have been on the right track. Later, we became aware of the benefits of electrically stimulating nerve pathways, but at that point, we were just beginning our learning curve.

All of the alternative therapies that Kathy tried had similarities. The most obvious was that they involved no drugs. The term alternative *medicine* doesn't actually make much sense since very little of it involves what most of us think of as medicine. We speculated that one reason the mainstream medical system doesn't pay much attention to alternative health care is because no dollars are exchanged with the pharmaceutical industry. We thought that was good. Kathy's goal was to rid her body of toxins, and pharmaceutical drugs were included on her list of things to avoid.

Another characteristic many of the alternatives had in common was that their treatments cost less than established medicine, but because they were seldom covered by health insurance, our out-of-pocket expenses were more.

For example, acupuncture treatments cost us between $65 and $100 per 60-minute session. A 20-minute visit to a general practice medical doctor cost $191 and a doctor-to-doctor consultation in the hospital was billed at $406. The insurance company paid the "real" doctor's bills without question, but refused to pay for Kathy's acupuncture treatment. One of the drugs prescribed for Kathy's ALS cost $1,003 per month, and it caused more problems than it solved. The natural potassium supplements that helped get her out of saliva hell cost about $14 per month, but the insurance company wouldn't even consider it.

Perhaps the most important characteristic of the alternative practitioners was their intent. Their goal was to assist Kathy's natural abilities to bring about healing, not to take over for her immune system. They wanted Kathy's body to be in charge. Their role was to help make that possible.

The care that Kathy received from established medicine was not about healing, it was about finding a cure. Instead of trying to improve her natural immune system through noninvasive means, the big league doctors prescribed drugs that made her immune system less efficient. That put her at the mercy of whatever the doctors decided to do. Without their benevolent intervention she had no chance of survival. Basically, it seemed like it was a matter of control.

Some of the alternative treatments that Kathy tried seemed a bit odd at first, but compared to killing off one's immune system, they were actually very sensible.

One of the stranger treatments that Kathy tried was an ancient Japanese treatment called moxibustion. It involved putting a small bit of the herb mugwort on the end of an acupuncture needle and then igniting the mugwort after the needle was in place. It put out quite a bit of smoke but had no visible flame. The mugwort burned at a specific, low temperature, which was transmitted through the needle. Kathy said that it didn't hurt or burn. I thought of it as a microscopically focused heating pad. Her moxibustion treatments were done at our home and had the side benefit of making the house smell pretty good.

Some of the alternative treatments Kathy tried had obvious benefits to her, especially the herbs, acupressure, massage and chiropractic treatments. Others may have assisted in slowing the progression of her disease, but there's no way to know for sure. None of the treatments did any harm. All of them gave her hope that healing was a possibility.

In November of 2006 we met Dr. Robert Waters, who runs a small integrative health clinic in Wisconsin Dells, about two hours away from Eau Claire. He is an MD with an open mind who believes that many of the alternative treatments have merit and should be integrated into the practice of medicine. He was the first person to take a look at Kathy's blood tests and recommend dietary supplements and vitamins to help restore her body to a more normal state. He also analyzed a hair sample and noticed an unusually high level of copper. The fact that the element showed up in her hair could mean that her body was ridding itself of excess copper. But where was it coming from? I took a sample of our household water to the county health department for analysis. The report came back with an attached warning sheet, alerting us to the fact that our water had unsafe levels of copper. We wouldn't have known that without the hair analysis. In January of 2006 I replaced all of the copper plumbing in our house and had the water retested. It was fine, however Kathy used only distilled water after that, which we distilled ourselves in the basement.

Perhaps the most important role that Dr. Waters played was as a knowledgeable person to react to and interpret the things that we continued to learn in our research. We visited him every couple of months and Kathy always brought along a list of her latest questions and discoveries for his opinion. He also reported to us about the latest things that he had learned from his research and from discussing Kathy's situation with his colleagues.

When Kathy found something that helped, he rejoiced with us. When we had questions, he helped us find the answers. We always felt better when we left his office than when we arrived.

Of course, insurance never paid a cent toward his bills, either.

CHAPTER TWENTY-ONE
Put Your Hands Behind Your Back

Thursday afternoon, Nov. 8, 2007. After lunch, Kathy decided that it was time to do her stretches. To keep her muscles from atrophying, she regularly did a series of arm and leg motions. A month earlier, when her albumin levels indicated she could begin trying to rebuild muscle, she added very light weights. Over the past year, her arm muscles had weakened considerably. She began having problems with her legs about the end of summer. For her legs, especially, the muscles still seemed quite strong, but accessing those muscles when needed was a different story.

Earlier that fall I had read about progress in rebuilding nerve pathways for people with spinal cord injuries. The idea was to *think* through a specific process as it was being done.

That reminded me of a study I'd read years earlier about pianists developing proper finger techniques. That study showed that pianists were able to improve their finger skills by spending time *thinking* through the proper movements without actually sitting down at the keyboard.

We had been working only on Kathy's arms and legs. We needed to include her brain, so we came up with a new approach that was sort of a combination of guided imagery and patterning.

For many months, when we did her daily stretches, I had

been moving Kathy's arms for her so that she could stretch beyond her own range of motion to keep her muscles from tightening up and atrophying. That helped keep them limber, but had no effect on improving her ability to move them on her own.

In early October we added the element of her having to mentally participate in each and every motion as it was being done. Our goal was both modest and practical: to improve the nerve pathways to the specific muscles in her arms that she needed to pull up her pants. We devised a set of seemingly simple motions specifically designed to trigger the muscles involved in that task. Each motion mimicked a movement she needed to pull her pants up to her waist.

First, we did a simple arm lift to warm up. I would stand in front of Kathy, at arm's length, take her hand in mine and she would extend her arm straight out and try to raise it to my shoulder, without bending her elbow. While doing this, she had to make sure that she didn't lift her shoulders.

As her arms had gotten weaker, she had developed a habit of using her shoulders to lift her arms, instead of actually trying to use her arm muscles. That was causing pain in her neck and shoulders.

When we began these new stretches, she couldn't raise her arms anywhere near as high as my shoulder, even with my help. When I tried to raise her arm that high it hurt and wouldn't move, as if the joint in her shoulder had rusted up. I also needed to support her arm at her elbow in order for her to keep it straight.

After less than a month of doing these exercises, I no longer needed to put my hand under her elbow; she built up enough strength to keep it straight on her own. She had also regained enough range of motion that she could hold her hand on my shoulder without my support and without pain.

Once her hand was on my shoulder, she had to hold it there and I would massage her arm from her wrist to her shoulder. If she let her arm fall off my shoulder while I was doing the massage, we'd start again. We did this for both arms and then began the pants-pulling exercises.

The first exercise was a simple crossing of her arms in front of her. She moved her right arm across her torso to touch the left side of her waist. Then she crossed her left arm over to touch the right side of her waist. It sounds easy, but she couldn't do this on her own without using a swinging motion to get the added boost of momentum. Once she swung her arm up to her waist, she couldn't hold it there; it would just drop back down.

We decided to outlaw swinging her arms. I would loosely hold her hands in mine, and when I felt her start to move her arms, I would assist. If I didn't sense her initiating the movement, I wouldn't assist and nothing would happen. With each motion, she would concentrate on sending the signal from her brain to her arm.

As she did this, I would tell her if she should move her right arm or her left arm. We figured that would force her to stay with it mentally. I also changed the pattern to force her to think harder about what she was doing. Right. Right. Left. Right. Both. Left. Both. Right. I needed to feel her beginning each movement before I would help.

After a few minutes of that, we'd move on to the next motion, which was to lift her arms from a straight-down position up to her waist. To practice this, she stood with her arms hanging straight down at her sides and I stood behind her and cupped my hands under her fists. This was the motion that we figured would be best to help her pull up her pants and had to be revised a couple times. I discovered by testing it out myself that when I pulled up evenly with both hands at the same time, my pants didn't come up very easily. To get my britches up, it was pull a little with the right hand, then pull a little with the left, in sort of a back and forth motion. So that's the motion that we tried to duplicate.

At first she tried to do the lifting with her shoulders. She had to concentrate on bending her elbows, instead. When I felt Kathy begin to lift her hands, I helped her raise them, an inch or two at a time on each side, until we got to her waist. Then she had to reverse the process and push my hands back down. She had to consciously start and stop them a little at a time all the way up and down. Sometimes, to help her keep her brain focused on her actions, I called out right or left and she'd do the motion with that arm. Other times she'd take charge and I'd have to pay close attention to which arm she was starting to move.

The next motion started out the most difficult for her, but became her biggest triumph. This one involved bending her arm up behind her back. At first, even with my help, she wasn't able to get it any higher than her tailbone without pain. That went on for more than a week until one day she concentrated especially hard and focused everything she had on the movement and it went right up to the middle of her back. Her range of motion didn't improve little by little. It suddenly went from almost none to full range. Triumphs like that are what kept us going.

This behind-the-back motion came along really well. As with the other exercises, when I felt her begin to lift her arm, I would help. It wasn't long before her arms didn't feel as heavy to me when I helped her raise them. One day, I decided to try a little experiment. After we did 10 lifts, I asked her to keep her hand up against the middle of her back while I let go. It dropped down immediately. She wanted to try again. This time she was able to hold it up for five seconds.

We got in the habit of timing how long she could hold it up every day. We went from five seconds to eight to 11 to 15 in five days. After a couple weeks we were at 60. On the Thursday that we went to see Dr. Sterner, in spite of how tired she was, she held each arm up for 65 seconds and could have gone on longer, but I called time.

We were both amazed at the progress she had made. Because we had been timing it, we could see exactly what kind of progress she was making. There was no question that she improved both her arm strength and control during the month that we did the exercises. She still didn't have the strength to pull up her pants, but we were seeing a definite and steady improvement.

The last motion was usually Kathy's chance to show off. We would place a straight-backed chair in the middle of the room and she'd sit down and lift her legs. I'd take a foot in each hand and try to spread her legs apart. I could almost never do it. I kidded her that it was because of her Catholic school upbringing. Then she'd relax her muscles, spread her legs and I'd try to push them back together. I did better on that one, but not by much. She'd alternate between open and closed without telling me, and enjoyed my frustration at being such a wimp. Her legs were always as strong or stronger than my arms.

Kathy said many times that she didn't want to lose her biking legs. She fully intended to be back out on the bike trail, riding her trusty Cannondale. I was amazed at how strong her legs were, but dumbfounded by how difficult it had gotten for her to direct those same legs to get her up the stairs.

That Thursday, after we did the pants-pull exercise, she said that she didn't want to do anymore. She wanted to skip the leg exercise. She was just too tired.

Showing me up with her leg strength was usually the most fun part of the routine—for her, at least.

Thursday, Nov. 8, 2007, was the first time she skipped it.

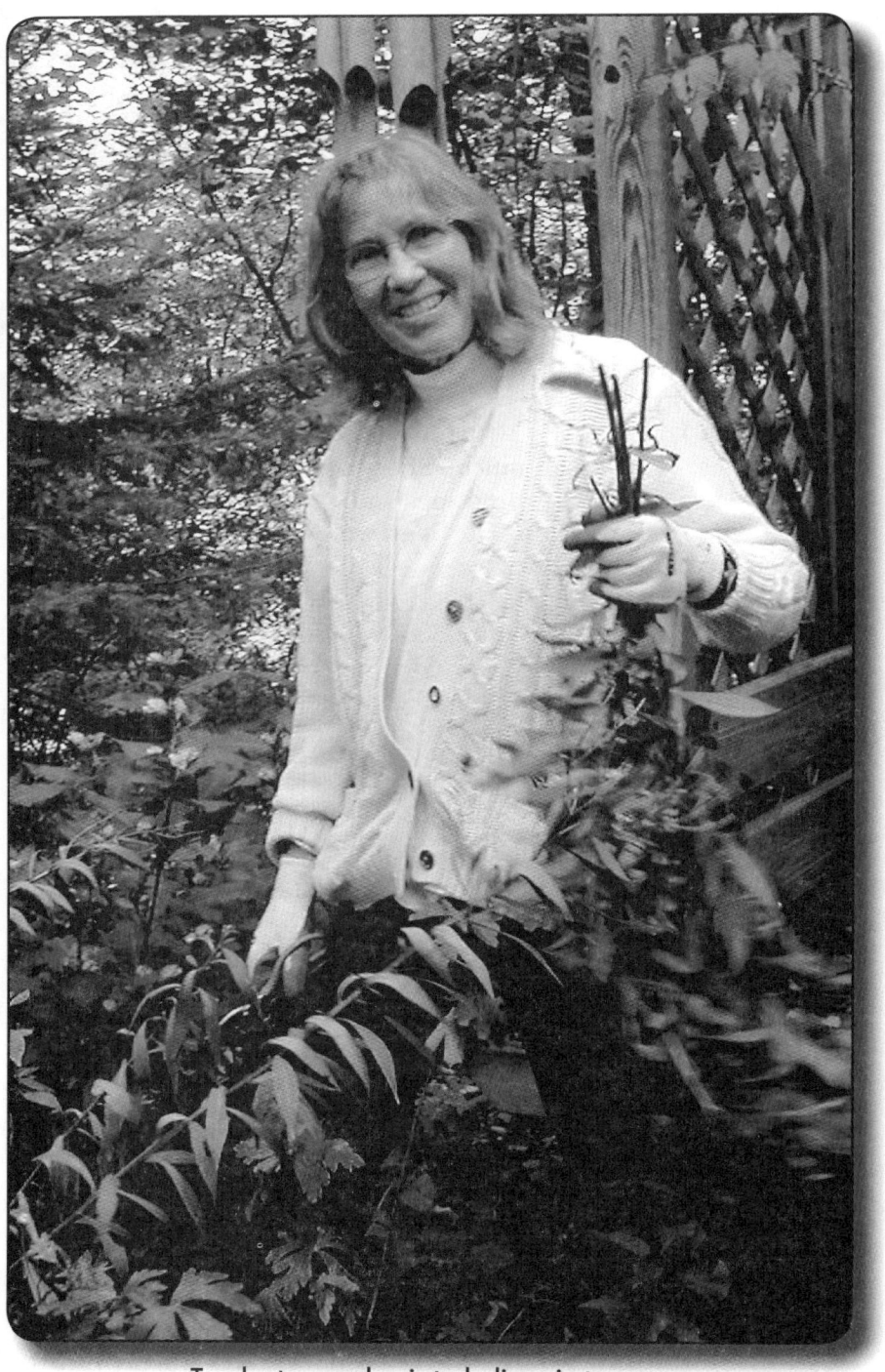

To plant a garden is to believe in tomorrow.

CHAPTER TWENTY-TWO
Garden Tending 101

Kathy loved gardening. I swear that she knew every one of the plants in our yard as a close personal friend. Six years ago she started her own garden tending business. In a typical summer she tended the gardens of about 25 families and a couple of businesses.

As she learned about the possible link between neuromuscular disease and environmental toxins, she wondered if garden chemicals may have contributed to her illness, especially when she discovered that ALS is especially common among farmers. She never used pesticides or chemical fertilizers herself, but she had no control over what her customers may have put on their gardens before she got there.

By the summer of 2006 she was able to care for only her own gardens, which were quite extensive. Even though her ability to garden was diminished, she found other ways to fulfill her gardening passion.

Since she had more time, she redirected some of her botanical passion to garden photography, which was something she had always had an interest in. She bought a light-weight digital camera, which was easier for her to maneuver, and chronicled her gardens from her point of view; close and intimate.

Most of her pictures were amazing close-ups that often included the little critters that shared her plants with her, such as insects, spiders and frogs. She was delighted each time that she met "someone" new among her flowers. If she photographed something especially fascinating, as soon as she came in the house she'd grab my hand and sit me down next to her computer so that I could enjoy what she found.

Throughout 2006 she posted pictures of what was blooming each month on her web site as a way to share her gardens with others. At the end of the 2006 season, she selected 52 of her favorite photos and made them into a perpetual desk calendar, which she gave to family and friends for Christmas.

Kathy also spent time researching and writing feature articles about gardening for the local newspaper. Sometimes she would pick a topic that she didn't know as much about just to give her something new to learn. When she wrote about starting plants indoors from seeds, we ended up putting together a tiny hothouse in the basement so that she could be certain that what she was telling her readers actually worked. She also wrote about her mistakes, as evidenced by a 2007 article about plants that she wished she had never planted. Somehow she always managed to find something positive about her adversities. In an e-mail to her editor she wrote:

> My garden is full of butterflies. Every day it seems I spot a new one. I had caterpillars gobbling up my cone flowers and rudbeckia, but I toughed it out and let them chow down to their heart's content. I like to think I am being rewarded now.

By the summer of 2007 Kathy's arms were too weak to do much digging or pruning, so she asked me to help her with much of the gardening. That was very brave of her. I wasn't much of a gardener—I had no need to be, living with The Garden Tender. We developed an interesting approach to gardening as a team.

In the past, my gardening duties included digging up new beds, hauling mulch and building and maintaining the garden structures. She was in charge of everything that was alive. It was a good arrangement: I knew little about plants and she had no interest in building arbors.

The biggest problem we encountered when I started helping her was with the plants that I didn't have a clue what I was doing. She had the knowledge, but because she couldn't speak she had a difficult time teaching me the difference between the sprout of a weed and her favorite perennial. Trying to write everything down on her white board was too tedious. So we worked out nonverbal cues.

A typical session would go something like this: first, she'd let me know what we'd be doing, such as planting, pruning, mulching or weeding and select the proper tools for me to use. Then we would head out together with the garden cart and wheelbarrow to a particular garden of her choosing. To keep me from being overwhelmed, Kathy usually had me work in only one section of the garden at a time.

Let's assume that we were weeding. When we got to the garden, she would take a long stick and point to a particular plant. I would touch the plant to make sure it was the correct one and she would then give me a thumbs up (it's a good plant... mulch around it) or a thumbs down (it's a weed... pull it out.) Once we got a rhythm established we could make pretty good progress.

One afternoon we were moving along particularly well in the bed along the picket fence, at the front of the house, the bed most visible to her from her office window. I was feeling pretty confident that I could tell the difference between a weed and a flower.

As she ran the stick up the stem of a fairly tall plant, I quickly snipped it off, without first touching it or looking for her signal. For a woman who could not speak, she let out a pretty loud shriek. She wasn't indicating that the taller plant should be removed, she was lifting its leaves so that I could see the weeds growing underneath. Instead of eliminating a weed, I'd cut off one of her most-prized dahlias.

That was the end of my gardening for that day.

Kathy could spend hours on end tending her gardens, but two hours was about all that I could handle at a time. The amount of help she needed varied with the weather and the growing cycles of the plants. Sometimes she could use my assistance every day, other times maybe only once or twice a week. She continued to do as much as she could herself, and only asked for my help with things that were simply too difficult to do alone.

On the days that she wanted my assistance, I usually found a note in the morning, saying something like, "Could I have 2 hours of garden time today, please? :-)" She added the smiley face to tasks that she thought I didn't particularly enjoy doing.

One of the first tasks of the growing season was planting her dahlia bulbs. There were boxes of them. Every fall she dug them up, overwintered the bulbs in the crawl space of the basement, and then replanted them in the spring, often in different locations. She had hundreds of bulbs, all carefully sorted and marked for color and height.

We planted the bulbs together in the spring of 2007. The bulbs were planted throughout the gardens, some in large groupings, others individually. She knew the color and size of the bloom that each bulb would produce. She knew which of the bulbs would grow tall and need stakes. She knew which needed the most sun. She kept track of some of this in her head, but much of it was written down in the gardening logs that she compiled at the end of the each season. It was a good thing that she painstakingly kept track of which bulbs she put into each box or bag the previous autumn, because to me the bulbs all looked pretty much the same.

Over the years, she had been carefully cultivating some impressively tall dahlias. When we started replanting them, she told me that the five-foot stakes I bought last year—the tallest ones available at the garden center—were too short. Just because something wasn't available from the usual sources, didn't mean that there wasn't another way to get what we needed. We replaced the five-foot stakes from the garden center with seven-foot tall stakes fashioned from furring strips. It took a bit more effort, but our homemade stakes worked better and cost half as much.

Throughout the summer, we worked together. She figured out what to do and when to do it, then stayed by my side to guide me through the tasks that took arm or hand strength.

As the summer ended, Kathy took careful notes about each of her gardens, highlighting the things that worked and jotting notes and questions about things that didn't turn out as planned. She did this every year.

The traits that Kathy used in tending her gardens—being organized, keeping track of her successes and failures, figuring out alternative solutions when needed—carried over into the way she managed her disease. She kept track of what she was doing. She knew what did and didn't help her. If the experts didn't have an answer for her, she was eager to look elsewhere for a better solution.

In late October of 2007 we began the process of once again digging and sorting the dahlia bulbs. She did that herself the previous year, but this fall I did all of the digging. Since I had helped plant them in the spring, I had a pretty good idea of what to expect.

Kathy directed me to each plant's remains and used a stick to point out where I should dig. She knew the exact location of each plant and what color and size it was, even though the only traces that remained were brown stems and shriveled leaves. The ones that were tied to poles were easy to track down, but only she knew the location of many others.

Using the system that we developed earlier, she pointed and I dug. As I dropped each bulb into a box or bag, she made a note on it indicating the flower's color and size. As we dug more bulbs, each would go into the appropriate container.

When we got to the spot where I had chopped off her special dahlia earlier in the season, I was a little nervous that she'd remember what I had done. She pointed to a bare spot on the ground and indicated that I should dig. I was relieved to find a bulb under the soil. I'd get a chance to redeem myself next summer.

That late October day, when we first began to dig up the dahlia bulbs, we spent nearly two hours working our way through the various beds in the front of the house. A year or two earlier, Kathy alone would have been able to complete all of the beds in the same amount of time it took the two of us to do the front yard.

The first week of November 2007, we spent another couple of hours digging bulbs. That day we finished many of the beds in the back yard. It wasn't as much fun that day. Kathy's energy level was much lower and it was getting colder outside. That day it felt like work.

On Thursday, Nov. 8, Kathy left me another note: "We have 2 finish digging dahlias today." Behind the words, two smiley faces.

Between my going to the clinic that morning, grading papers and finishing some other small tasks, it was already late afternoon by the time I was ready to dig bulbs. It was chilly outside, only in the low 40s. The night before it had gotten down to 29. It wouldn't be long before the ground was frozen and Kathy was concerned that the remaining bulbs would be ruined.

I helped her put on her coat and we headed out to the last of the gardens, at the very back of the yard, next to the tree house. All of those dahlias had been tied up on stakes, so they were easy to find. Once we had the boxes organized, Kathy wrote, "I'm 2 tired 2 stay out here. You'll go faster without me, anyway."

It wasn't like her to walk out on her plants.

She pointed out the colors of the various plants, showed me which boxes to put the bulbs in, then went inside. She had never left me alone in her gardens before. Either she had come to trust my skills or she was exhausted. I wanted to believe the prior, but I knew it was exhaustion. I had a little extra energy because this was the day after Ann had spent the night. But Kathy's energy levels continued to fall as her sleep deprivation became more severe.

It had been suggested to her a couple weeks earlier that she take melatonin supplements. Melatonin is a naturally occurring hormone that helps to regulate sleep. It seemed like a good idea and I bought a bottle at the health food store, but when Kathy researched it she discovered that while it was generally regarded as safe for most people, it was not advised for people with auto-immune diseases. She asked me to return it to the store, unwilling to risk winning the skirmish with sleeplessness, but in the process, losing the war against her ALS.

When I finally finished digging the bulbs it was getting dark outside. Kathy looked glad to see me come in. She was sitting at the computer writing to daughter Emily:

> Hi babe,
>
> i;m notdoing so great.having a hard time holding mt head-up. met a newdoc toda y. she prescribed ph ysical therapy to b uild up backmuscles alsolooking 4 so m eon e   who can do vit c iv w ee kl y. david got las t of dahleas out few minutes ago. whew!
>
> last night ann s ta yed ovver so david couldge t sleep.
>
> lovingu,
>
> momXXOOOxx

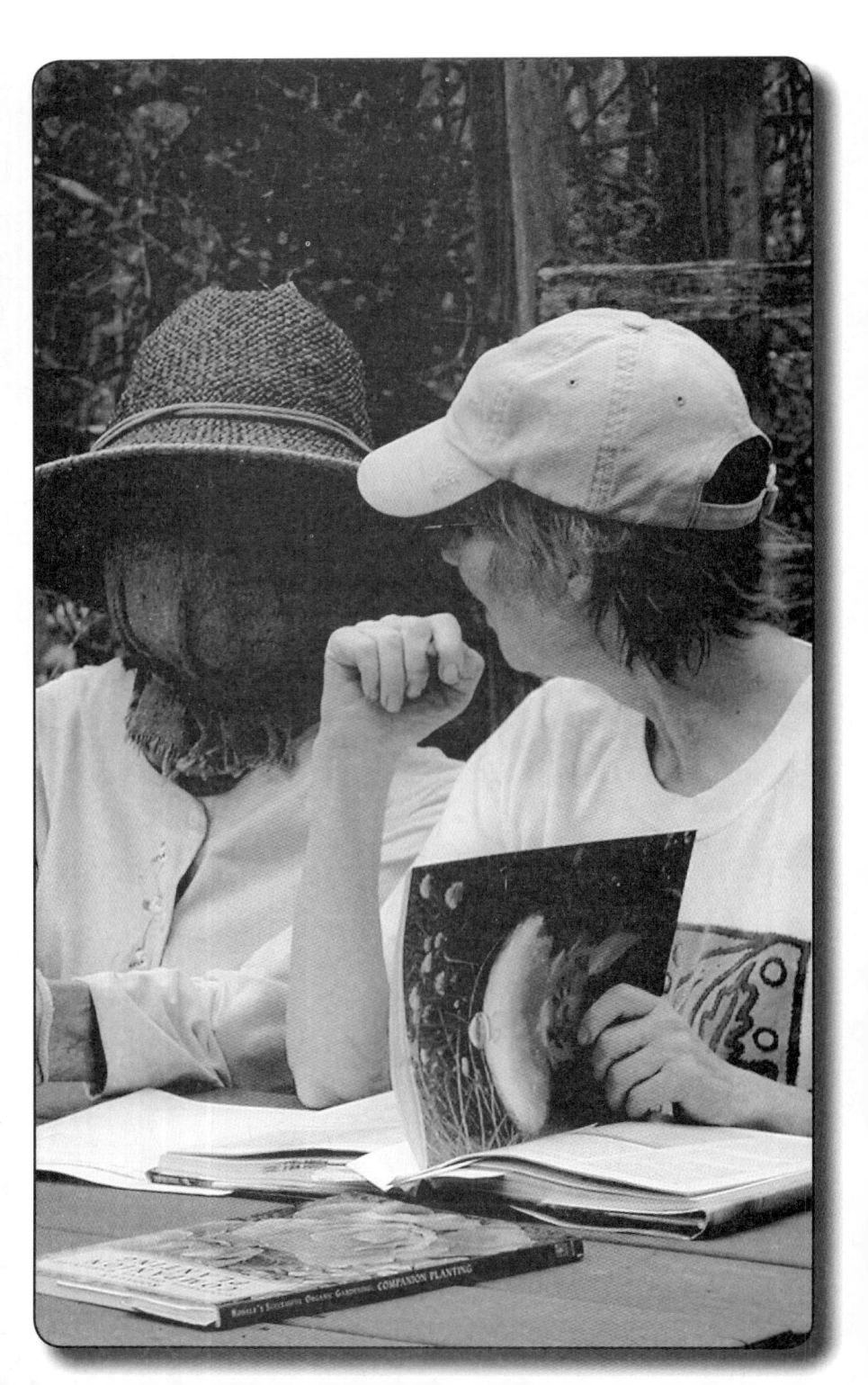

CHAPTER TWENTY-THREE
Berry Picking in Bayfield

Kathy's sister once asked me, "Is it possible for Kathy to ever just sit and do nothing?" My answer was easy: "No."

Having to "do nothing" while I made supper each evening was frustrating for Kathy. We had always taken equal roles in meal preparation and she enjoyed cooking. She had a reputation for being extremely good at baking pies.

Her specialty pie was made with tart cherries that we picked in Bayfield, Wisconsin. Every year we would drive up to that lake-side community to pick cherries, raspberries and blueberries. After we finished picking, we would enjoy a meal of Lake Superior whitefish. Then we'd take a stroll through the scenic little town and treat ourselves to a hand-dipped ice cream cone. It was a day-long vacation that we looked forward to every summer.

Our last trip to Bayfield, in August of 2007, didn't turn out so well. We hadn't taken any extended day trips since we returned from Texas. It was simply too much work to pack up everything needed for Kathy's meals and too big of a concern that she might choke on her saliva while we were driving.

But when we received the summer newsletter from the berry farm saying that they'd soon be picking blueberries, we decided to give it a try. We were desperately ready to do something fun, and adding some blueberries and raspberries to our diets would be okay since they weren't exotic fruits. We had gone to the same berry farm for a number of years and recalled talking with the grower about the natural ways that he kept pests off of his plants.

We decided against picking cherries, because we knew they weren't organic and reaching up to pick them would be impossible for Kathy.

Before we could go, I had to prepare some meals for Kathy. I packed two jars of blended food, one for lunch and one for supper, and an extra in case one was spilled or we had car trouble and needed more meals than expected. We couldn't simply stop at a restaurant or grocery store and get the food that we needed. Even if we could find a way to blend it up, it wouldn't be organic or include the right mix of ingredients and supplements.

The jars needed to be kept cold while we traveled, then warmed up before the meal to get the food thin enough to go through the tube. At home that was easy. We'd simply set the jar in a bowl of hot water for 30 minutes. That didn't work on the road.

We found a small travel cooler that plugged into the cigarette lighter. It could also function as a food warmer, depending upon which way you set the switch. We started the day with it set to cool. About an hour before mealtime we stopped and switched it over to heat the food. The extra jars of food were kept in a separate small cooler with ice packs.

It was a very good thing that the truck had air conditioning, because it turned out to be a very hot day, in the 90s. Kathy seemed especially bothered by the heat.

We stopped once or twice on the way to Bayfield so Kathy could use her tongue scraper to pull the phlegm from her throat and get a drink, using the syringe. She couldn't trust her sense of thirst. On a sweltering day like this, when she knew she'd need extra water, she had to keep a close eye on the clock.

The berry farm was more crowded than normal when we arrived. It was a great crop, with lots of large berries on each tiny bush, which would make for quick picking.

As we pulled into the parking area, I asked the farmer, "Are your berries grown organically?" It had become a habit to double check almost everything to make sure that it was free of chemical pesticides and herbicides.

"We use all natural farming practices," he assured us. I was about to pull forward when I noticed Kathy writing "Is it organic?"

"We're not certified organic," he said. "But we do use only sustainable practices. You can pull ahead and park next to those other cars."

Some organic farms don't seek official USDA organic certification, even though everything they do is organic. But I could tell by the look on Kathy's face that his answer wasn't good enough. "Pesticides?" she wrote.

"Do you use any pesticides on your berries?" I asked.

"Only once in the season, at the very beginning," he answered. "Never when there's any fruit."

That was not the answer we wanted to hear. Chemicals sprayed on the blossoms tend to stay in the fruit. Even if it was an extremely small amount, any risk at all was more than Kathy was willing to take. We had driven 180 miles, were looking at the blueberries and couldn't pick them.

Then we recalled passing a sign for an organic farm just down the road and decided to check it out.

The organic farm wasn't visible from the road, but after traveling a short distance down a wooded, curving driveway we came to a place straight out of a Foxfire book. Instead of long rows of blueberries and someone directing traffic, this tiny farm had a little bit of everything, all sort of jumbled together. They also had only one customer.

After a little searching, we found the owner and he assured us that they used no pesticides or herbicides and were certified organic. This would do.

Unfortunately, the blueberry bushes that he had were larger and the blueberries were smaller, making them much more difficult to pick. He gave us a couple of milk crates to sit on and directed us to two blueberry bushes, a few yards apart, which he wanted us to pick clean. Instead of easily reaching down to pick handsful of berries, as we could have done at the other farm, here we needed to maneuver our hands through the branches. As we sat on the crates, many of the berries were higher than our shoulders. In the hot sun, it was a lot of work. Because the bushes we were picking weren't together, we couldn't even see each other to keep tabs on how we were doing or give each other a wink. There wasn't room for us to work together on the same bush.

Every little while I walked over to see how Kathy was doing. At first, she was picking faster than I was. But as she had to reach higher, she began to slow down. After about 30 minutes, we each had picked only half an ice cream bucket of blueberries, far fewer than we'd have picked in the same time at the other farm. None-the-less, we decided to call it quits. It was too hot and too much work.

"Should we still pick some raspberries?" I asked.

She shook her head. She'd had enough and wanted to go home.

We walked back to the truck, hand-in-hand, carrying our buckets of berries, looking like an older version of the cute little kids in bibs and gingham who often showed up on our anniversary cards. I suspect, though, that we didn't have their same smiling faces. That hot August day in Bayfield, we felt defeated.

On the way home, we needed to stop for gas and a bathroom break. Finding a suitable bathroom was no longer an easy thing to do. The rest rooms in the larger convenience stores have multiple stalls and no locks on the main door. That didn't work very well since I needed to go in with Kathy to help her with her pants. Usually, I helped her get situated in the bathroom, then went back out and stood guard at the door until I heard a knock on the wall, indicating that I should come back in to get her.

Once, at an Interstate rest area, the main door to the women's rest room was propped wide open, so I stood in the doorway, leaning against the frame. A couple of women came up to use the bathroom, saw me standing there, and walked away. A minute later, they came back and I told them that I was waiting for someone and would be going back in to help her. They gave me an annoyed look and went back out to their car and drove away. I hope they didn't need to go too badly, because the next rest area was more than 100 miles down the highway.

On our way back from Bayfield, we stopped at a small, locally owned station. The bathrooms weren't particularly clean, but we had the place to ourselves. I went in with Kathy and got her started, then waited outside the door. When I heard her knock, I went back in to help her pull up her pants. She was feeling pretty tired, so I walked back out to the car with her, then came back to pay the cashier.

"I'd have been happy to take your wife into the bathroom so you wouldn't need to go in there," she said politely as I paid the bill. "I'm trained as a first responder and know how to deal with people who are disabled."

I believe that the woman meant well, but she just didn't get it. It was hard enough for Kathy to have me take her into the bathroom. The last thing she wanted was to be accompanied by a total stranger.

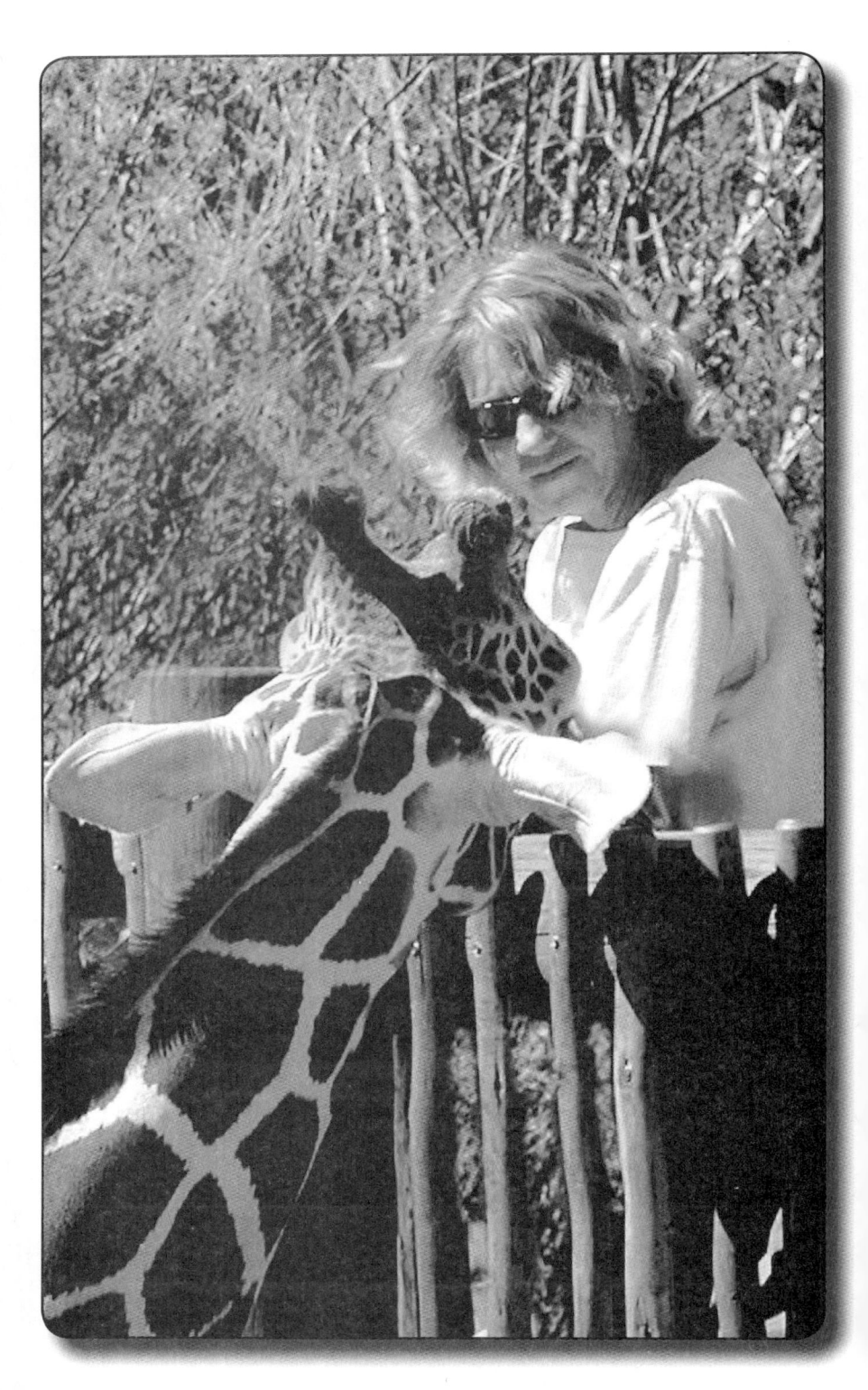

CHAPTER TWENTY-FOUR
Fourteen Times and Counting

On Thursday nights we usually watched "CSI" and "Without a Trace." We had watched those shows for a long time and, like almost all of the television programs that we enjoyed, we watched them together, sitting on the couch. That Thursday, the day we visited Dr. Sterner, there was a special, combined episode of the two shows, with the characters from the two programs intermingling.

Sometimes we recorded the earlier of the two shows so that we wouldn't be so rushed, but that night we wanted to watch them in sequence, which meant that we'd need to shower quickly.

After our shower, we noticed that Kathy's weight was continuing to increase. She was up to 115, a pound and a half heavier than she was a week earlier. It had gone up a little each of the last few days. We thought that the weight gain may be from the water retention in her ankles and feet.

The previous day, we sent an e-mail to Doc Huggins asking him if he thought that the salt in her diet may be the cause of the water retention. He responded: "Go ahead and reduce the salt intake because she may be approaching saturation even thought the blood does not indicate it." So we cut back on the salt by 50 percent, from 4.5 teaspoons per day to 3 teaspoons per day. We hated to do that because at the 4.5 level her saliva was controlled and she could function quite normally, without constantly drooling.

As we'd feared, within a day the amount of saliva increased, not to the point that it had been when she was in saliva hell, but enough to once again be a nuisance, especially when she was trying to sleep.

We finished with our shower duties just in time for the beginning of the two-hour "CSI/Without A Trace" big event. Sometimes we had to get excited about the little things in our life.

During the first hour of the show, Kathy sat next to me so that I could massage her neck and shoulders. Jodi, the chiropractor, had told us the day before that I should start massaging the muscles on the front of Kathy's neck and on her upper chest in order to help her lift her head more easily. About half an hour in the front seemed to help, so I switched to the spot on her left shoulder that continued to give her the most discomfort.

I had started massaging that spot almost three weeks earlier, within hours after she'd hurt it by falling in the kitchen. At first it was quite a knot, but it seemed to be improving. The visits to Jodi helped, as did regular treatments with heating pads and ice packs. But it still caused a lot of pain when she tried to rest or sleep.

By the time we got to the second hour of the television program, I told Kathy that we'd had enough of this "official" massaging for the day; it was time for a foot rub with massage oil. Nothing relaxed her more than having her feet rubbed. So she lay back onto her nest of pillows, her feet on my lap, and we made believe she wasn't sick, that we were doing this because we wanted to, not because we had to. I don't recall any details about the television show. But I very clearly remember the two of us together on the couch, relaxed and enjoying each other's company.

The night that followed, however, was anything but relaxing. As usual, it took a long time to get settled into bed. The night before, Wednesday, when Ann stayed over, Kathy got up during the night only six times. In terms of the number of times getting out of bed, Wednesday was a very good night. But she had gotten very little sleep.

On Thursday she was up 14 times, about every 45 minutes. Sometimes she got up to use the toilet. Sometimes she got out of bed to use the suction machine to deal with the newly increased flow of saliva. Sometimes she got up simply to could get back into bed from a different angle so she could sleep on her other side.

In the middle of all that, without any warning, she once again wet the bed. So, in the wee hours of the morning we found ourselves standing in the bathroom with a soapy washcloth, searching through the dresser for a clean pair of pajamas, and figuring out how to put enough towels over the bedding so that it wouldn't soak through before morning, which we hoped would come quickly.

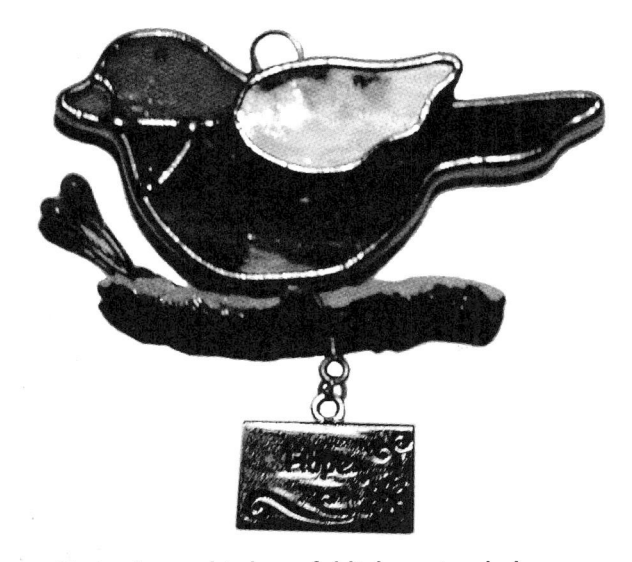

Kathy hung this hopeful little stained-glass sun catcher in the window next to her desk.

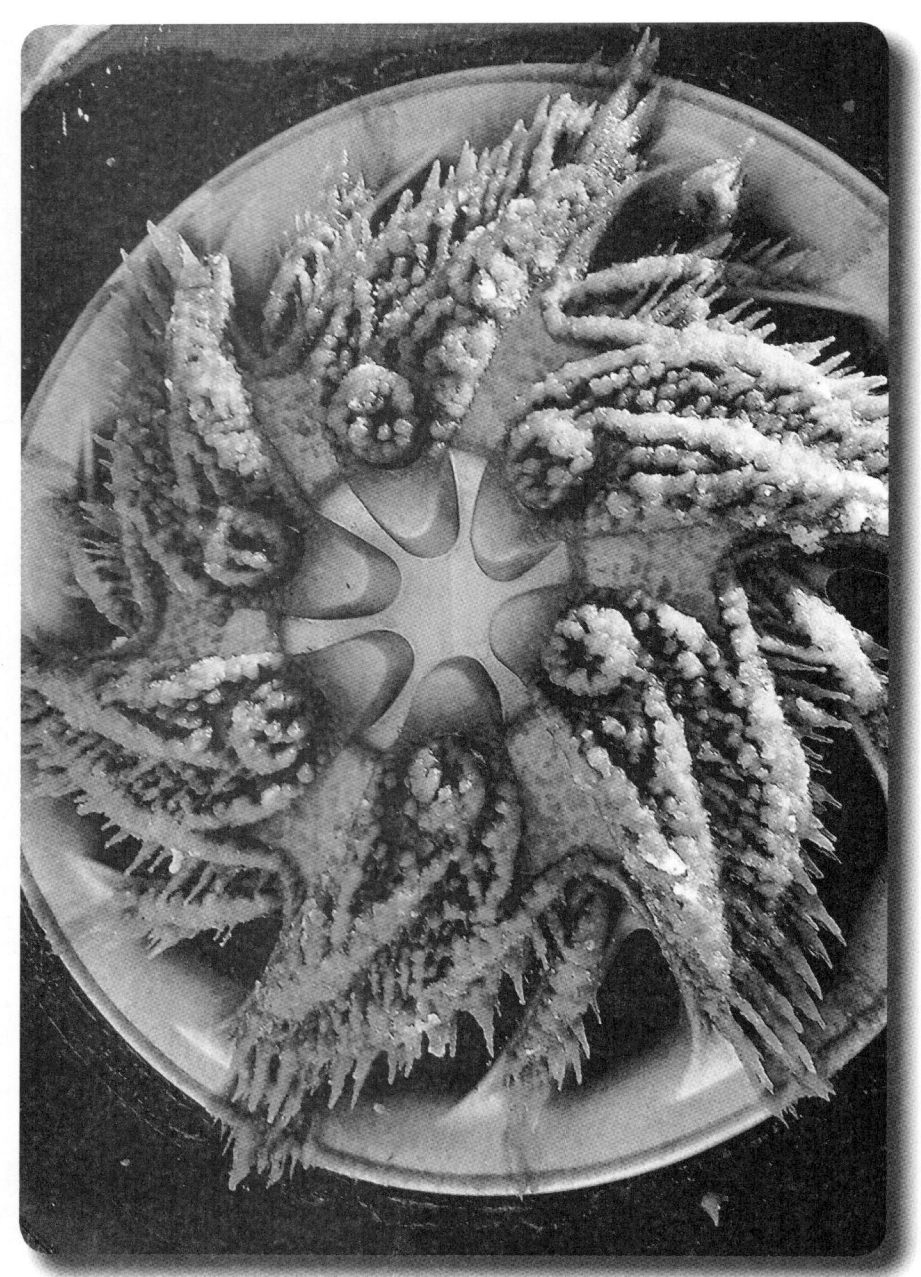

In January 2007 Kathy got caught in an ice storm on her way home from a chiropractic appointment. I was at work, worried about her safety. When she arrived home, she took this picture and e-mailed it to me. Instead of complaining about the horrible drive, she found beauty in the pattern that the ice had formed on her tires.

CHAPTER TWENTY-FIVE
Friday, Nov. 9, 2007

The day began with phone calls and e-mails in search of someone who could help Kathy with the vitamin C IV. I followed up on a lead and discovered a doctor in town who worked in a chiropractor's office doing chelation treatments. I talked with him by phone and he was able to set up the IV, but he wasn't willing to come to our house. I told him that we had the exact instructions for the procedure from the clinic in Texas, and he said that he would decide for himself the best way to set it up. He answered a few more of my questions rather grumpily and never even asked about Kathy. Comparing that conversation to some of the other calls I'd made in the past, I decided to look a few other places before scheduling the appointment with him. I wanted to make sure that he was going to be supportive of Kathy in her pursuit of healing, not just treat her as another paying customer. Personal support was essential to her healing.

After Kathy was diagnosed with ALS, she received some get well cards, as might be expected. It seemed obvious that many of the senders had done some quick research on ALS and learned that it was always fatal. Most of the get-well cards were pretty weak on the "get-well" part.

One of the cards, though, made Kathy feel awful. She described it as "a sympathy card sent while she was still alive." The card and the handwritten note inside reassured her that she had nothing to worry about because she would soon be with Jesus and have a new body in heaven. I'm sure that the sender's intentions were good, but Kathy felt that she had been written off as dead. That was not the message she wanted or needed to hear.

After she decided to beat the monster inside of her, she had no intention of being held back by the negative attitudes of people who did not believe she could do it. She wanted to surround herself with people who would be a positive influence, people who would encourage her, people who would root for her recovery.

After that "sympathy" card, she asked me to open and read every card and note she received and discard those that were negative. There were several that she never saw and at least one that I wished I hadn't seen either.

Still trying to figure out someone who could set up the vitamin C infusion, Kathy thought of a friend who taught at the local nursing college. Perhaps she could help us arrange something, maybe with a student. The woman was out when I called, so I sent her an e-mail:

> Do you think that any of your students would be interested in working with Kathy on this? They could set it up and then study over here until it was done. We have wireless access, so that would be handy for a student needing to be online. Plus, it'd be great experience in patient care.

Kathy also recalled that a friend's wife was a nurse or medical technician and wondered if she may have some leads or be able to do it herself. Kathy sent an e-mail:

> The reasoon i'm writing is i 'm goin downhi ll fast. we're trying fi nd a nurse to co me 2 th he huse 2 set me up w/a v it. C iv. Wondered if U knew someone.

Then we were off to the chiropractor's office for the third appointment of the week with Dr. Jodi Swartz. Kathy's neck and shoulder felt better after each of the first two appointments and she was looking forward to going back for further treatment..

The part of the treatment that Kathy appreciated the most was the electric stimulation. Kathy asked Jodi to turn it up as high as she could to get the most benefit.

As promised, Jodi had checked to see if a similar machine was for sale locally so we could do the treatments at home. She reported that she hadn't found any. I had located a couple on e-Bay and she gave me some tips on what to look for before buying one. The biggest problem with buying an electric stimulation machine on e-Bay was that I would need to wait for the auction to end, and until then I wouldn't know if I would actually get it. The process could take a couple of weeks. Kathy needed the machine now. She couldn't go on much longer with so little sleep.

Kathy asked Jodi if she would be willing to come to the house sometime for a treatment. Jodi said that she'd be happy to if she could work it into her schedule. It was always easier if we could figure out a way to treat Kathy at home, both in terms of time and convenience. Before we left the office, Jodi wrote down two dates and times on the appointment card and we headed home.

In early October, Kathy asked Ann if she would come over to help her with a few household tasks, such as dusting and washing furniture. Kathy felt bad that nearly all of the chores were falling on me and was quite sure that I'd never get to some of them on my own. Ann agreed to come over on Friday afternoons while I was at school. I appreciated that. I also felt more comfortable knowing that Kathy wouldn't be home alone, especially after her fall in the kitchen.

That Friday afternoon, though, Kathy asked Ann to massage her neck instead of help her clean. They talked again about the value of humor therapy and enjoyed each other's company.

About an hour before bedtime, Kathy tried an herbal sleep aid. She was desperate for sleep and when one of her friends suggested an herb called valerian she immediately researched it. She couldn't find any downside to it, so she asked me to pick up a bottle on the way home from work.

One whiff of the stuff made us both rethink the wisdom of putting it into her body. It smelled like old silage. Because Kathy couldn't taste her food before putting it into her body, she had to rely on her sense of smell (and my pre-tasting) to know if it was spoiled or good to eat. We found a little magnet with a picture of a fox eyeing a skunk and placed it prominently on the refrigerator door. Under the picture were the words, "If it smells bad, don't eat it."

The recommended dose of the green powder was three capsules before bed. Because it smelled so bad, she decided to be cautious for the first try and had me give her only one capsule. A good thing. Within an hour she had a stomach ache, which made her sleep even worse.

That night Kathy was up at least a dozen times. Around 2 a.m. she started kicking at the covers, trying to get them off of her. I pulled them back, thinking she wanted to get out of bed. She kept kicking. I could hear her taking loud, short breaths. I helped her sit up. By this time she was hyperventilating; breathing in and out very rapidly, maybe two breaths a second. We didn't have a routine for this, so I began rubbing her shoulders and neck, trying to calm her down. After a few minutes, her breathing began to return to normal. After another 15 minutes of my rubbing her neck she calmed down, but still couldn't relax. She decided to try some meditation techniques she had recently learned and finally, after about 30 minutes, was able to lie back into her nest of pillows. I pulled the covers back over her.

Within moments I could tell by the tensing of her body and the sound of her breath that she was on the edge of another panic attack. I had no idea what to do to stop it from happening, and finally said, "Kathy, do you remember the night we walked along the Pacific Ocean and it was so foggy we couldn't see anything, but we could hear the waves next to us?" She indicated that she remembered. "Do you remember how peaceful that was? How calming? Let's make believe that we're there now." I took her hand as if we were walking along that invisible beach and started making sounds like waves rolling up onto the shore. Amazingly, it helped. We both fell asleep.

For a few minutes, at least.

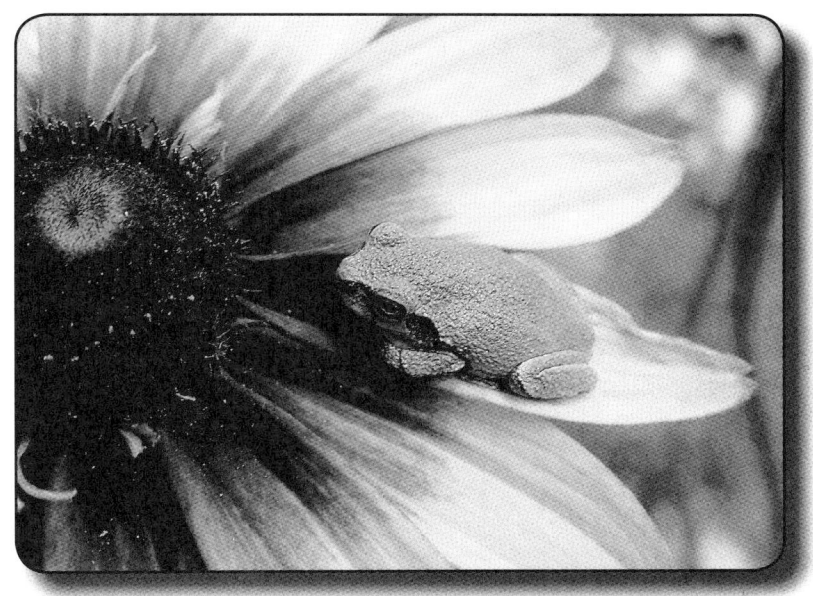

This little frog, no bigger than my thumbnail, was one of Kathy's favorite photo subjects.
—*Photo by Kathy Tank*

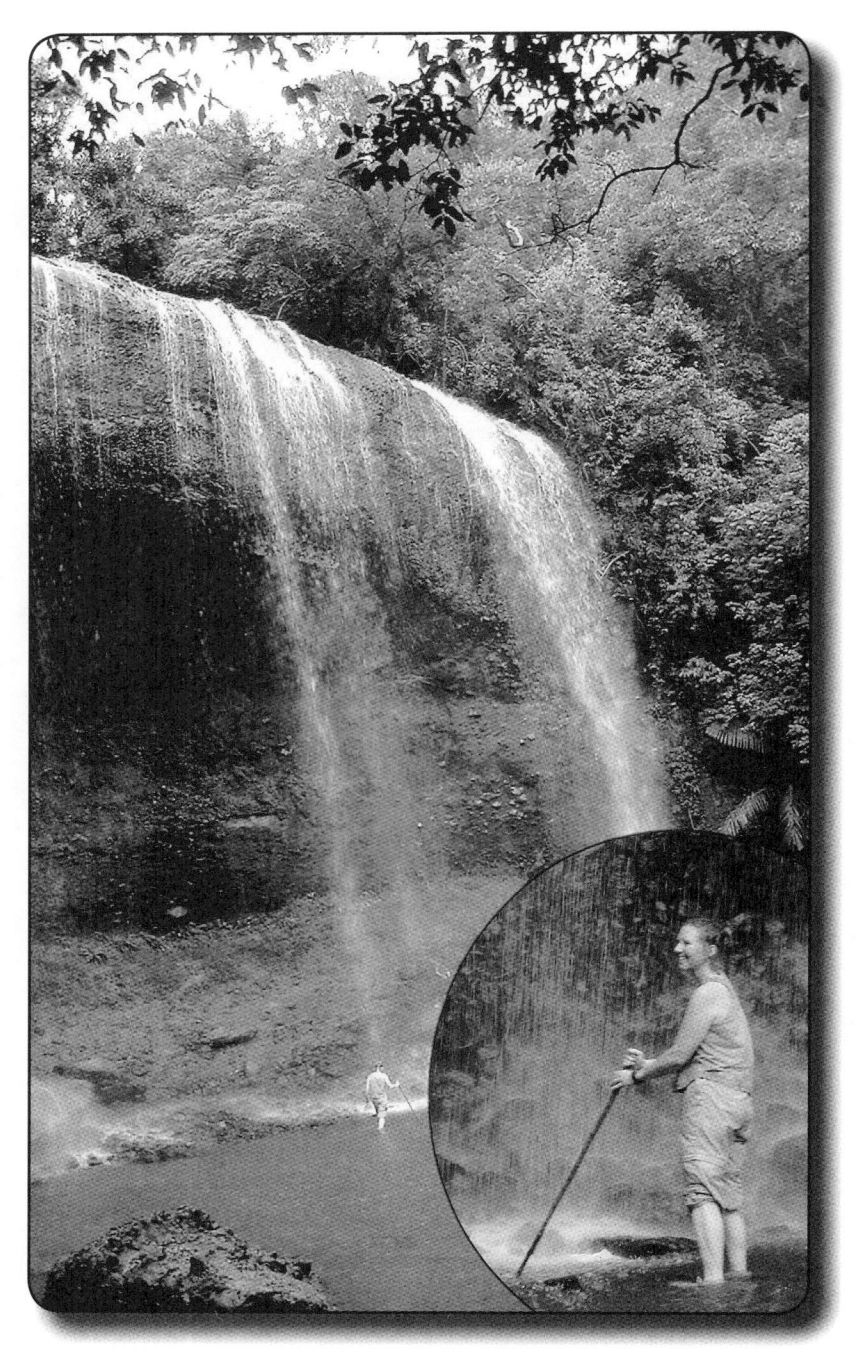

CHAPTER TWENTY-SIX
Saturday, Nov. 10, 2007

We started the day by once again washing sheets and pajamas. Perhaps imagining the sound of waves in the night wasn't all that good of an idea. Kathy hadn't told me when it happened, not wanting to burden me with the extra middle-of-the-night tasks involved if I had known.

Saturday afternoon was daughter Hilary's baby shower, about 90 minutes away in Minnesota. Hilary had talked with Kathy about coming to it a month earlier, but Kathy didn't think she'd be able to attend. Hilary told her at the time not to say "no," because maybe by the time of the shower, she'd be feeling better. Obviously, she wasn't.

We talked about having some flowers delivered to Hilary's house, but Kathy decided that wasn't a good idea because mass-produced flowers are heavily sprayed with pesticides and fungicides and she didn't want to put Hilary and her unborn child at risk. She said there were still a few flowers in her gardens and she'd like to make a bouquet of them to send to Hilary, if we could figure out how to get them to her.

It occurred to me that my mother and sister would be driving quite near our house on their way to the shower. They said they wouldn't have any extra time to stop, though. It was a six-hour drive for them from southeastern Wisconsin to Minnesota.

That was probably okay. We were already running late. Then the phone rang. It was my mother calling from the road. They started earlier than expected and said they could stop by to pick up the flowers in about half an hour. That was great, except for one thing: we didn't have any flowers ready for Hilary.

Kathy and I quickly headed outside. She grabbed a pointing stick and I grabbed the clippers. Fortunately, Kathy knew exactly where the surviving flowers were and which ones she wanted. She pointed them out and I clipped them off. By the time my mom and sister arrived, a small bouquet of hand-picked, autumn flowers was ready for delivery.

One of the items on my To Do list for the day was to build the compost pile. Most of the soil in Kathy's gardens began as leaves, grass and kitchen waste. She had composting down to a science and for many years handled that project entirely on her own. The past summer, we built and turned the compost piles together. She determined the correct ratio of leaves to grass clippings, and I mixed the components together while she added water from the garden hose. We still had a lot of leaves and clippings to put into the compost bins before winter. Kathy told me that this time I would have to do it alone. Even though it was a pleasant day to be outside, she said that she was too tired. She'd stay in the house and try to take a nap.

By the time I finished, she still hadn't been able to get any rest. She'd spent most of the time reading a book about ultra longevity, and moving back and forth between the rocking chair, couch and dining room table. Tired as she was, she simply could not sleep.

She added a new item to my To Do list: Would I go to the store and buy a package of disposable absorbent underwear that she could wear to bed. Because I knew she didn't like being home alone, I grabbed her sweatshirt, assuming she'd go to the store with me. She said that she didn't have the energy to go along.

"Hurry," she wrote on her white board.

When I came back, she was sitting in the sun porch, reading about a new gardening technique she was planning to try in the spring. As always, the radio was on to the classic rock station. I barely got my jacket off when she cranked up the radio full blast. Out of its speakers blared the song "Start Me Up," by the Rolling Stones. That was our cue to start dancing. We'd done it a million times in the past year. Whenever "Start Me Up" came on, we stopped whatever we were doing and danced around the house as if we were Mick Jagger and Keith Richards. Usually she was Mick and I was Keith.

This little game began early in 2007 when Kathy was finding it more and more difficult to lift her arms over her head. She wanted to figure out how to build them back up and knew from her experience with aerobics, that she could coax more from her body with the addition of a good, strong, musical beat. The song "Start Me Up" came on the radio and she thought that worked very well. She casually mentioned this to her brother, Gary, who e-mailed a YouTube video of the Stones performing the song live. There at the front of the stage was Mick Jagger, stabbing his arm high into the air with each beat. It was perfect. She decided it would be fun to do this dance together.

So every time "Start Me Up" came on the radio, we would break into spontaneous dance. After a while, Kathy recorded the song and left it in the CD player so whenever she got the urge she could hit play. No matter where I was, in the basement, at my desk or out working in the garage, when I heard the opening chords to "Start Me Up" I was expected to join Kathy and start dancing.

Sometimes I would hit the play button and she'd have to stop what she was doing and join me. A couple of times, on especially nice days, we cranked the stereo as loud as it would go and danced our way outside, weaving through the gardens. If the neighbors saw us, they must have wondered if we'd gone insane. One time the song came on over the speakers while we were shopping. We looked at each other: "Should we?" We refrained... but just barely.

As Kathy grew more and more tired, trying to raise her arms in time with the music became more and more of a struggle, more and more discouraging. Neither of us had hit the play button in several weeks.

But when "Start Me Up" came on the radio just as I returned from the store, Kathy couldn't resist turning it up. Even though we were both exhausted, we got up and danced. We may not have danced as well as Mick and Keith that afternoon, but we had fun, something that had been missing from our lives for awhile.

Saturday night was no improvement over Friday night. It did help that Kathy didn't have to use the toilet, but she was still up eight or 10 times to change position, plus she went into the bathroom a couple of times to get a drink or suction out the saliva.

Each time she tried to get back into bed, it got more difficult. It often took three or four tries for her to get up onto the mattress. After one failed attempt she slid off the edge of the bed and onto the floor, where she lay exhausted until I lifted her back into bed.

I placed a little stool next to the bed, thinking that would make it easier for her the next time she got up. The idea was sound, but she wasn't able to lift her foot onto the six-inch stool. Earlier that day we had been dancing to "Start Me Up." A dozen hours later, she couldn't lift her foot more than a few inches. The rest of the night, whenever she needed to get into or out of bed it was a two-person job.

There was one positive side to the night. By wearing the absorbent underwear Kathy was less tense, knowing that if she had an accident, it wouldn't be a problem for both of us. In spite of the sleepless night, we got up the next morning more relaxed.

CHAPTER TWENTY-SEVEN
Sunday, Nov. 11, 2007

On Sunday morning, when I helped Kathy get dressed, she said she wanted to try wearing the disposable unders during the day. She figured it would give her a bit of a safety net in case she had any problems, especially since my mom and sister would be stopping for a longer visit on their way back from the shower and I might not be easily available to help her in the bathroom.

I usually go out on Sunday mornings to get a newspaper, but Kathy didn't want to be left home alone and didn't feel up to going along. That surprised me. The latest gardening article that she'd written was scheduled to be in that Sunday's paper. It was about gardening books to read in the winter, when you are trapped inside and looking forward to spring. I knew she was curious to see which pictures they ran with the article.

Several weeks earlier, her sister and brother-in-law came to help prepare her gardens for winter, and she convinced them to pose for a picture, sitting in the rocking chair reading a gardening book. Neither really wanted to do it, but she convinced both of them to give it a try and she'd let the editor decide which one to use. She was eager to know which he'd chosen.

Even so, she preferred that I stayed home with her. I could get the paper later. She was feeling restless again. I helped her get comfortable in the rocking chair to read and put the ice pack on her shoulder. She'd been using the ice pack regularly, often alternating it with the heating pad, as recommended by the chiropractor. She was eagerly awaiting her visit with Jodi the next morning. The pain in her neck and shoulder had gotten much worse since her last visit on Friday.

Once I got Kathy settled into the rocking chair, I lifted her legs up onto the footstool. A couple of minutes later I heard a thump. It was the sound of her feet falling off of the footstool onto the floor. I walked over to her, lifted them back up. "Please try to stay in one place longer than 10 minutes," I said. I didn't want to sound bossy, but I could tell that moving around so much wasn't doing her any good. I was hoping that maybe, if she could stay in one place for awhile, she would fall asleep and get some rest.

The 10 minutes lasted maybe nine. Once again I heard the thump of her feet falling off the footstool. By the time I got over to her, she was trying to get out of the rocker, but she couldn't get quite enough momentum to make it up. "Just stay there," I said and lifted her feet back onto the stool for the third time. I had barely turned around when I heard the thump again. If Kathy didn't want to do something, she wouldn't. I think she also enjoyed teasing me.

I put my hand under her arm, tipped the chair back, then rocked it forward and said "one." I rocked it back, then forward a second time. "Two." Back and forward again. "Three." With the extra rhythm and momentum Kathy was able to stand on her own without needing much of my assistance.

Of course, that didn't solve the problem of where she'd go next and how long she'd stay there. She headed for the couch and after about five minutes of rearranging the pillows was ready to try taking a nap. That lasted about five minutes, as well. She simply could not get comfortable.

Next, she decided to sit at the table in the porch to read. She often sat out there, but for the past couple of days she hadn't been able to scoot the chair in on her own, so I pulled it out for her, she sat down, and I slid it back under the table. The old wooden school chair did not slide easily on the carpet and I didn't have the strength to simply lift the chair. Fortunately, she stayed there, reading one of her gardening books from the library, for about 30 minutes. Then she was ready to move again.

This time it was to the table in the dining room. Once again, I pulled out the chair, she sat down, and I slid it under the table. That was especially difficult for me in the dining room because the rough berber carpet made it harder for me to slide the chair with her sitting on it.

Not many days earlier, I noticed a chair that might make my job easier. It was similar to a regular wheelchair, but smaller, without foot rests or big back wheels. It seemed like it might work well for sliding Kathy in and out from under the tables. She could probably even do it herself. I wasn't sure, though, if I should even mention it, recalling her earlier, negative reaction to my proposal to buy a regular wheel chair from the resale store.

"Kathy," I said, "I saw a really cool chair that I think would make it easier for you to read at the table without needing my help." She seemed interested, so I described it. To my surprise and relief, she agreed that it might be a good idea and said that I should buy it the next time I was out.

Before she had a chance to move again, my mother and sister stopped in on their way back from Hilary's baby shower. Kathy seemed especially happy to see my mom. The two of them always got along great and had many interests in common. They chatted in the corner by themselves, my mom with her voice, Kathy with her white board.

One of the things they talked about was Kathy's plan to help Hilary with a quilting project. She and Hilary had been planning it since summer, but it was put on hold when Kathy lost the strength in her fingers and couldn't work on it. Now, Kathy was optimistic that her hands would improve enough by winter to resurrect the project, especially with Sarah planning to come by twice a week for acupressure and massage treatments. Kathy sensed that her body was ready to take another step forward, if only she could get some sleep.

Sometimes her progress came as a surprise. A couple weeks earlier I arrived home from school and walked in the door with my usual, sappy, "Hello, Honey, I'm home." Often, she would make some sound of acknowledgement, but it was usually so soft that I could barely hear it from the back door. But that evening, instead of a soft sound from the living room, I heard Kathy call back "Hello." I could hear her just fine. The word was still slurred, but it was obvious that she had said "hello."

I went around the corner to take off my shoes and called back to her, "Wow, I could hear you all the way by the back door. You've got a lot of power in your voice tonight. You must be feeling pretty good."

From close behind me, came four words: "I know, I am." I turned quickly. Kathy was standing behind me, smiling.

"You just said, 'I know, I am!"

"I know," she answered, but not quite as clearly.

I don't know if she'd been practicing, waiting for me to come home, but she looked as surprised and excited as I was. That was definitely a huggable moment. She didn't try saying anything else the rest of the evening.

That night, after we were in bed, she tried speaking to me again but I couldn't understand her. She repeated it, but I still couldn't make out the sentence she was trying to say. After seeing how happy she was earlier, I felt awful that I couldn't understand her, but I didn't want to guess—I learned early on that was a bad idea—and asked her to repeat it one more time. She shook her head and slurred the word "no." I asked if she wanted me to get her white board. She indicated no, squeezed my hand and we tried to fall asleep. That was three or four weeks earlier, shortly before her fall in the kitchen.

After my mom and sister left, Ann came over to stay with Kathy while I went to a meeting of the regional ALS support group. Kathy and I had heard about the group's existence not long after her diagnosis. But after the gloom-and-doom experience we had in Madison, Kathy said that the last thing she needed was to be around more people who were convinced that she would die. She didn't want to learn about wheelchair ramps and cough machines. She wanted to talk to people who would help her get better.

The reason we finally decided that I should go to the support group meeting was because we needed information about home health care in the area and figured that the folks in that group would be able to tell us who was good and who to avoid. Kathy did not want to go along.

The ALS support group, which met in a church, seemed like a small group of friends. Two of the people had ALS. Two others had spouses who died of neuromuscular disease, but stayed active in the group. The leader, a woman named Deb, welcomed me and made me feel at home.

After a brief discussion about some videos that were available and a couple of items of new business, including the upcoming Christmas party, they introduced their guest speaker. It's a good thing that Kathy stayed home. His presentation was about the ventilation equipment ALS patients will need when they can no longer breathe on their own. He also promoted the cough machine.

The presenter held up a huge mask and explained that in order for the ventilator to work correctly, the face mask needed to fit snugly over the person's mouth and nose. If it didn't fit tightly, it wouldn't work. I asked how someone would get it off if she started to choke, but couldn't lift her arms as high as her face. He acknowledged that would be a problem.

Someone in the group brought up that the ventilator they used was very noisy, and wondered if the new ones were quieter. He pointed out that the newer ones were less noisy and that after five years Medicare would allow you to buy a new one, as long as the old one was no longer working.

Since he was a specialist in assistive equipment, I asked if he knew anything about suction machines and explained that the one we had didn't work and wondered if it could easily be fixed. He asked a few questions to see if I was setting it up properly. I was quite sure that I was correctly following the instructions. He said that he could look at it.

Then I mentioned that I had built my own suction machine for $30 from a one-gallon ShopVac. He was not particularly impressed and expressed his concern that it was probably dangerous. That made me a bit defensive. I pointed out that it worked great and that the expensive one didn't work at all.

Someone in the group asked about getting rid of an oxygen machine that was no longer needed. The presenter pointed out that it could not be thrown away because of some disposal rule and it could not be given away or sold because that could only be done with a prescription from a medical doctor, and the doctor's orders would only be good for a new machine, not for a used one. In other words, even though there was a perfectly good machine available and there was a person who needed it, it was against the rules to pass it from one person to the other.

When I made a crack about it sounding like the health care supply business was being run by some sort of medical mafia, the speaker decided it was about time to wrap up his presentation. *Oh great,* I thought, *the first time I come to the group and I insult their guest speaker.* I figured I'd better get out of there, too.

After he left, one of the people in the group commented that I seemed rather anti medical establishment and wondered why. I told them about Kathy. The first part of the story was very familiar to them. Everyone present had been told about the hopelessness of his or her situation and had first-hand experience to back it up.

It was the second part of the story that started them asking questions. Mercury in dental fillings? Neurotoxins in pesticides on our foods? Drugs that destroy the body's immune system? I told them about the book "Eric is Winning" and about Doc Huggins' work with biochemistry. When I mentioned that Kathy had recently begun swallowing some water and feeling movement in her tongue, they wanted to know more. Not one of them had heard any of this before.

I also told them about Kathy's recent fall in the kitchen and her inability to get any sleep. They asked me to bring her along the next time I came to their meeting, as an inspiration to the group. I was afraid that my rant about the medical mafia was going to get me thrown out. Instead, it got me invited back with Kathy. People need hope.

Before I left the meeting, I learned something especially interesting. They mentioned that a member of their group had just been put into a hospice facility. He had been in a wheelchair for some time and was in the last stages of ALS, with very limited mobility.

His name caught my attention. It was a man who first showed symptoms of ALS at the same time as Kathy. She didn't know him but they had a mutual friend. The man's symptoms began the same as Kathy's, with difficulty speaking and swallowing. For the first year and a half, the disease progressed at the same rate for both of them.

When Kathy first learned about the man, she sent him an e-mail to see if he had any advice or suggestions for her. The note she got back reflected his total lack of hope. He had resigned himself to the fact that he had an incurable, progressive disease and would simply let it take its course.

It's not necessarily a good idea to try to compare this man whom I've never met, with Kathy. But their situations started out in the same way at the same time. Even their place of employment at the onset of the disease was the same. For the first year and a half, while he and Kathy both sought care from the medical establishment, their illnesses progressed at about the same speed. I learned later that after that, his disease progressed much faster than hers. When she was giving up biking because it was difficult to steer, he was moving into a wheel chair because it was difficult for him to move. When Kathy was again starting to swallow, beginning to feel movement in her tongue and getting a bit of strength back in her arms, he was being moved into a hospice.

I hated to learn that this gentleman was near death. It struck too close to home. On the other hand, it did seem to indicate that Kathy's efforts were paying off. Her disease had continued to progress, to be sure, but she was in much better shape than he was. Her biggest problem at the moment was her inability to get any sleep.

I thanked the group for their interest and went home.

Since it was Sunday night, it was time for another soak in the tub. Neither Kathy nor I thought it was a very good idea. Kathy didn't think she had the strength to get back out of the tub and was afraid she'd be trapped there. I feared that she'd slip out of my grasp and get hurt. We decided to postpone it until the next night. She decided to sit on the couch and watch TV.

While she was sitting there, the phone rang. It was daughter Emily. In the past, whenever Emily called, Kathy would drop whatever she was doing to talk with her. Usually, I would chat with Em while Kathy went upstairs to her office and connected the phone to the voice synthesizer on her computer. From there, she could type what she wanted to say, and the computer would speak the words directly into the phone line. She used a headset to hear the other side of the conversation, which allowed her to use both hands for typing.

For more than a year, Kathy used that system regularly and usually successfully. But not recently. Her typing had gotten so poor in the past few weeks that the words spoken by the computer were often gibberish. She would need to type very slowly and carefully for the process to work. Emily was very patient, though, and Kathy always looked forward to her calls.

That Sunday night when Emily called I expected that

Kathy would ask me to help her up the stairs so she could take the call. Instead, she stayed on the couch, looked at me sadly and wrote, "Tell her I'll e-mail her."

I decided to talk with Em for a while and took the phone into the bedroom so I wouldn't disturb Kathy as she watched TV. After a few minutes, a Munchkin came walking into the bedroom. Kathy felt bad about not getting to talk with her daughter, but wasn't able to stand up when she tried to get off the couch. So she walked to the bedroom on her knees. It was hard not to laugh at how odd she looked.

Still on her knees, she placed her white board on the bed and wrote "Hi Em." I repeated the message, then put the phone to Kathy's ear, with my ear next to her's so we could both hear what Emily was saying. Kathy would write out her response and I'd read it into the phone for Em. It wasn't the greatest system, but it worked.

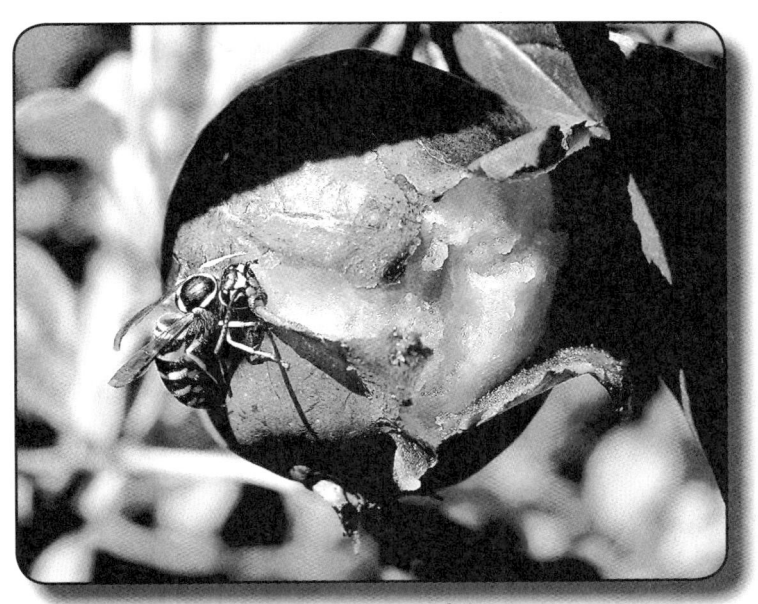

Kathy shot a series of pictures of this wasp eating a crab apple. She was fascinated to discover that it peeled the skin away before eating the flesh.

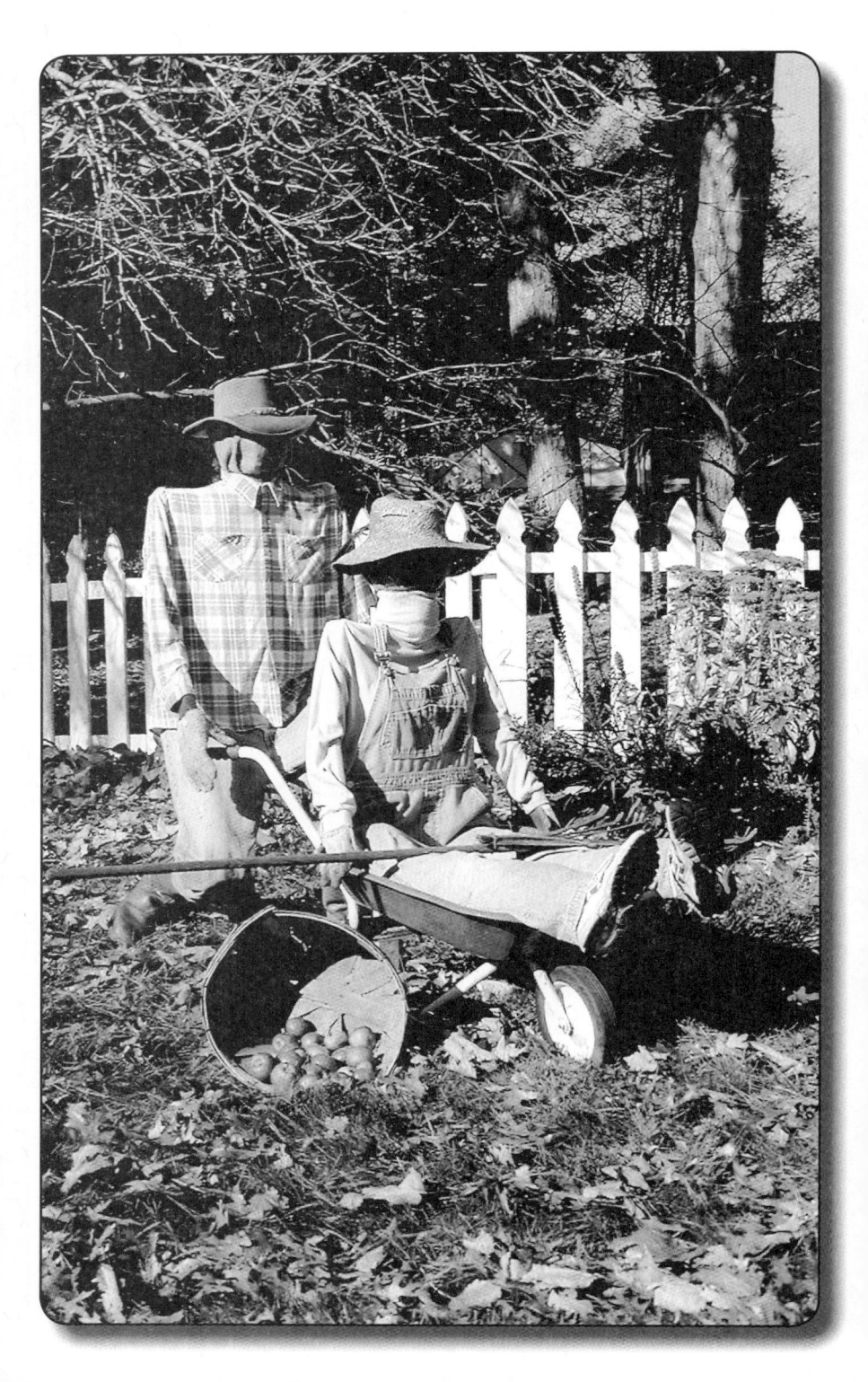

CHAPTER TWENTY-EIGHT
Monday, Nov. 12, 2007

Sunday night did nothing to help solve Kathy's sleep deprivation. If anything, she got up Monday morning even more tired than when she'd gone to bed. The constant ups and downs, ins and outs, with only a few minutes of sleep were rapidly taking their toll. She couldn't lift her head at all and had a hard time standing without her shoulders hunching over.

The bright side of the morning was that in a few hours Kathy would be getting another treatment from Jodi, the chiropractor. Throughout the weekend, the pain in Kathy's neck and shoulders had continued to worsen. I suggested that she try rubbing some pain-relieving cream onto her neck and shoulder, but Kathy said that wasn't a good idea. She said she'd checked it out and learned that it worked by affecting the nerve pathways. She didn't want to try anything that would reduce her nerve function.

She spent much of the morning reading her book on longevity. She had ordered it through interlibrary loan and it had to be returned in three days and couldn't be renewed. Her determination to finish it before it was due helped keep her sitting in one place until it was time to go to the chiropractor.

Kathy regularly made fun of how poorly I drove my manual-transmission Geo Metro. Jumpy and jerky was a polite way to describe it. That morning I tried especially hard to drive smoothly. With every bad shift, Kathy's head would bob and I could see her grimace. She didn't complain, but there was no question that she was ready for this appointment and the relief that it would provide.

We arrived at Jodi's office a few minutes early, shortly before 11. The lights were on, but the door was locked. We wondered if we were the first appointment of the day and expected to see Jodi coming to unlock the door at any moment.

After a few minutes, I knocked. No one answered. By 11:10, Kathy was having a hard time standing, even though she was leaning against the wall. On the other side of the glass office door we could see the waiting room chairs, but we had no way to get to them.

"Are you sure this is the right time for the appointment?" I asked. "Were we supposed to be here at 10?" Kathy was sure that it was the right time.

At 11:15, she said that she couldn't stand up any longer. We slid a sorry-we-missed-you note under the office door, then slowly walked back to the car. Since we now had some extra time, I suggested that we stop on the way home to look for a lower bed frame and a wheeled chair. Kathy wrote three words on her board: "Home. Ice pack."

When we walked into the house, the light on the answering machine was flashing. It was Jodi. She had been sitting in our driveway, wondering where we were. At the same time that we were leaving her office, she was pulling out of our driveway. We'd forgotten that this was the day she was coming to our house.

Kathy asked me to assist her with her pants in the bathroom. When she finally rang the bell for me to come back, she looked defeated. I held the water tube up to her mouth as she leaned over the sink so that she could rinse her mouth and feel the cold water run down her throat. That made her feel a little better.

After lunch I noticed a couple of comedy videos stacked

next to the TV. Ann brought them to watch with Kathy the day before, when I was at the ALS support group meeting. I asked Kathy if she'd like to watch any of them. No. She'd rather sit in the rocking chair with the heating pad on her shoulder. After 20 minutes, she switched to the ice pack for 20 minutes, then back to the heating pad, then the ice pack. The combination of heat and cold worked best to ease her pain. It also had the side benefit of keeping her in one place for more than an hour.

At about 3:30, I told Kathy that I was in serious need of a nap. She suggested that we take a snooze together in the backyard treehouse. The treehouse, with its reclining futon, was one of the few places where Kathy was consistently able to relax and get some rest. She enjoyed the sound of the water running into the pond and the music of the five-foot wind chime hanging in the tree.

"It's really cold up there," I said. "And I've already drained the pond for winter, so there won't be any sound of the water. We shoulda thought of it sooner so I coulda turned on the space heater."

She gave me her "you're doing it again" look.

When we were first married I had a habit of complaining that "I shoulda done this" or "I coulda done that" or "if only I woulda done something else."

"You've got to stop with the 'coulda, woulda, shouldas,'" she'd tell me. "Don't say you should have done something else. Instead say that the next time you'll do it differently. You can't change the past."

After a while, when I did a shoulda-woulda-coulda, she'd simply say "you're doing it again." Over time, that phrase turned into a simple, recognizable look. In the days and week to come, her insistence that I not bemoan the things I'd done in the past would turn out to be one of the best gifts she'd ever given me.

Since I'd shot down the idea of napping in the treehouse, I helped her build a pillow nest on the porch. Once she was settled in, I went into the bedroom and lay on the bed for a nap of my own. About 10 minutes later I felt her climb up next to me. Try as we might, neither one of us could get to sleep. Whenever she would start to nod off she'd begin to panic. I asked her why she was so scared. She wrote, "Don't no. Just get terrified." A little after 4, we gave up. Attempting to get to sleep had become more tiring than staying awake.

We went into the living room and flipped on the TV. I don't recall even once before watching daytime TV together. Maybe the change of pace would be good. We snuggled next to each other on the couch, her head on my shoulder, and watched "The Ellen Degeneres Show." Every once in a while we'd nod off, but never for more than a minute or two. Nevertheless, we considered the hour a success. It may not have been the naps we'd hoped for and needed, but it was restful, and the silliness of the program took our minds off of the predicament we were in.

Kathy's restlessness continued throughout the evening. She didn't want me to be out of her sight, so I worked on some school papers in the dining room while she watched "Heroes" and "CSI: Miami."

When we took our shower, she leaned her head against the wall the whole time and never even tried to lift the washcloth. Her weight had gone up four pounds in the past week, most likely from the fluid retention in her ankles and legs.

Neither one of us wanted to go to bed. We watched Leno for awhile, but finally surrendered and went into the bedroom. Once again, Kathy was constantly in and out of bed. As the night went on it became more and more difficult for her to get back into bed. One time while she was in the bathroom to use the suction machine, I got up myself. When I returned she was already back in the bedroom, on the floor next to the bed. Instead of crumpled against the wall, as I had found her two nights earlier, she was on her knees, like a little girl saying her prayers. Maybe that's what she was doing. She didn't look upset about being there.

Kathy was never a person to wear her faith on her sleeve. She didn't particularly like the rituals that went along with being a member of a church. More than once she told me that she liked what the church taught; it was the going-to-church part that she didn't much care for.

Earlier that fall I saw her standing in the kitchen, appearing to be deep in thought. When I walked up to her she wrote, "There are four churches praying for me." I knew that four different churches regularly included Kathy in their prayers for healing; our own congregation, her sister's congregation and the congregations of two friends.

"Do you like that?" I asked.

"Yes," she wrote. "They believe I will get better."

"Do you pray?" I asked.

"Yes," she answered, "but I'm sick of praying 'Your will be done.'"

"Then don't pray it," I said.

"That's what I was taught to pray. Are U praying?"

"I am" I answered. "Almost every time I wake up in the night."

"What do U say?"

"Lately, I've been saying, 'God, I'm getting really sick of You teasing Kathy; making her a little better at the same time other parts of her body get worse.' I've been telling God that He should quit fooling around and if He's so powerful, He should do one of His miracles and heal You.'"

"U R going to make God mad," she wrote.

The previous summer, Kathy mentioned to Joyce, a friend of ours, that what she craved the most was a simple drink of cold water. The next day, Joyce told her that she had made a promise to herself: every time she had a drink of water, she'd say a prayer that Kathy would be able to have a drink of cold water again, too.

About 3 a.m. we finally decided that since neither one of us was sleeping, we might as well get out of bed. We went into the living room, sat on the couch under one of Kathy's quilts, and watched the fish swim around in the lighted aquarium. We sat there for at least an hour, leaning on each other, holding hands, falling in love all over again.

At 6:30 we decided to get up for good. We weren't sleeping anyway and we had come to hate being in bed. It had been the worst night ever. Kathy was up at least 20 times. The longest stretch that she stayed in bed was 20 minutes, the shortest, eight. I don't think that she got any sleep at all. Whenever she'd close her eyes she'd begin to panic.

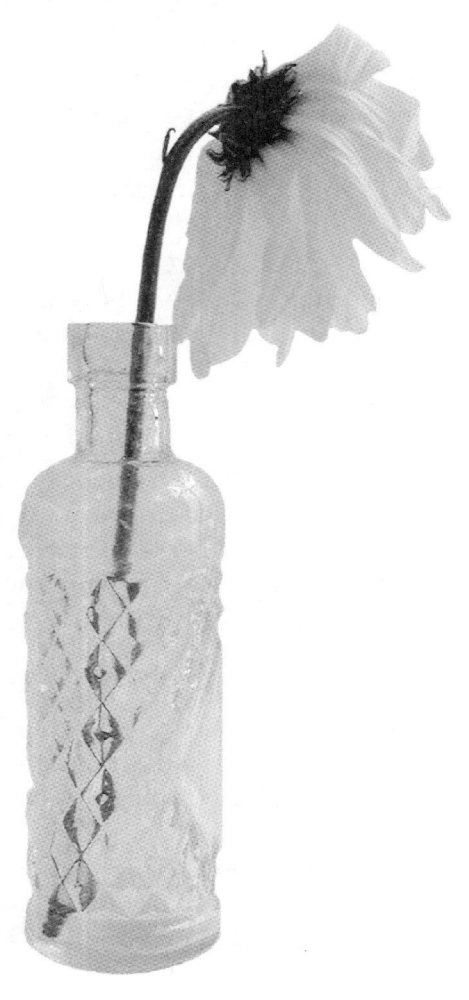

CHAPTER TWENTY-NINE
Tuesday, Nov. 13, 2007

I washed Kathy up in the bathroom and helped her put on a fresh pair of unders. She said she had no plans to even try to use the toilet; she had no control over it anyway.

Usually, Kathy picked out what to wear, but since she was so draggy, I decided to pick out some comfortable clothes for her. She rejected all of them and wrote on her board: "Look like a clown." Then she picked out others that she liked better.

She went in the living room and sat in her rocking chair by the window. It was the place that she could relax the best, a soft lap blanket folded gently behind her neck. She continued reading her book about living a long life; she was on a chapter about the value of biking and dancing.

I put together her usual breakfast, then went to get her. We did the one, two, three thing to her get out of the chair, but I could tell as we walked to the kitchen that instead of just walking hand in hand, she was relying on me to hold her up. That was unusual. I told her I was concerned she couldn't easily stand at the counter to eat breakfast and suggested that I bring breakfast to her. She agreed so I walked her back to the rocking chair.

Breakfast went well. The morning sun was shining in the front window. Even though she had great difficulty holding her head up, she seemed in good spirits. She tried using the cervical collar that we'd bought a week earlier, but she only kept it on a few minutes; it was too uncomfortable. That was always the case with that thing. She felt trapped in it. I replaced it with a couple of rolled up towels under her chin.

At 8 a.m. I phoned Ann and asked if she would come over and tell me what she had learned the night before at a care givers meeting she attended. I also wanted to see if she had any suggestions about what we could do to help Kathy get some sleep.

Ann arrived about 8:30, took one look at Kathy and said she thought that we needed to put her into a nursing home to get some sleep, and that we should do it that day. Kathy shook her head sideways, which was difficult for her to do, and wrote "no" on her board.

Quite a few months earlier, after a horrible choking spell, I was trying to find out from Kathy how she wanted me to handle an emergency situation. "Should I call the ambulance?" I asked.

"Maybe," she wrote.

"How will I know when to call?"

"Only if I am unconscious." Then she added, in all capital letters: "I WILL NEVER, EVER FORGIVE YOU IF YOU EVER, EVER LEAVE ME SOMEWHERE OVERNIGHT ALONE."

I promised that I would never leave her alone. Ever.

Now, as I stood next to the rocking chair trying to figure out what to do, I clearly saw that white board in my mind and my promise to her.

I asked what I could do to help her? She wrote something, but her hand was shaky and I couldn't read it, so she wrote it again. "Ice pack." I got an ice pack for her neck. After it was in place, Ann went behind the chair to help calm her, rub her shoulder, and help hold her head up to ease the pain.

I decided to at least find out what was involved with getting Kathy into a nursing home, but had no idea how to go about doing that. I decided to call Dr. Sterner, whom we had met the Thursday before, and ask her advice. She wasn't in, but I explained Kathy's situation to her nurse and was told that a triage nurse would call me back with a suggestion.

I went over to Kathy to tell her that I'd made the call and someone would be getting back to us soon. "Is there anything else I can do for you?" I asked. She wrote slowly, so I could read it the first time: "Help me sleep."

The triage nurse called me back almost immediately and after hearing what was going on, recommended that I bring Kathy to the Luther Hospital ER where they could put us in contact with a social worker and possibly get her into a nursing home.

I went over to tell Kathy and Ann what they'd said. Kathy had fallen asleep, her head in Ann's hands. She finally looked relaxed. She looked beautiful. I hated to disturb her.

"Kathy," I said, kneeling next to her and putting my hand on her arm. "We're going to take you to the ER so they can help you get some sleep."

She didn't respond.

"I think she stopped breathing," Ann said softly, almost as if she didn't want to disturb Kathy's calm.

"Kathy?" I gently shook her arms. She took two small breaths and that was it.

I checked her pulse. Nothing.

Without a moment's hesitation, I dialed 911.

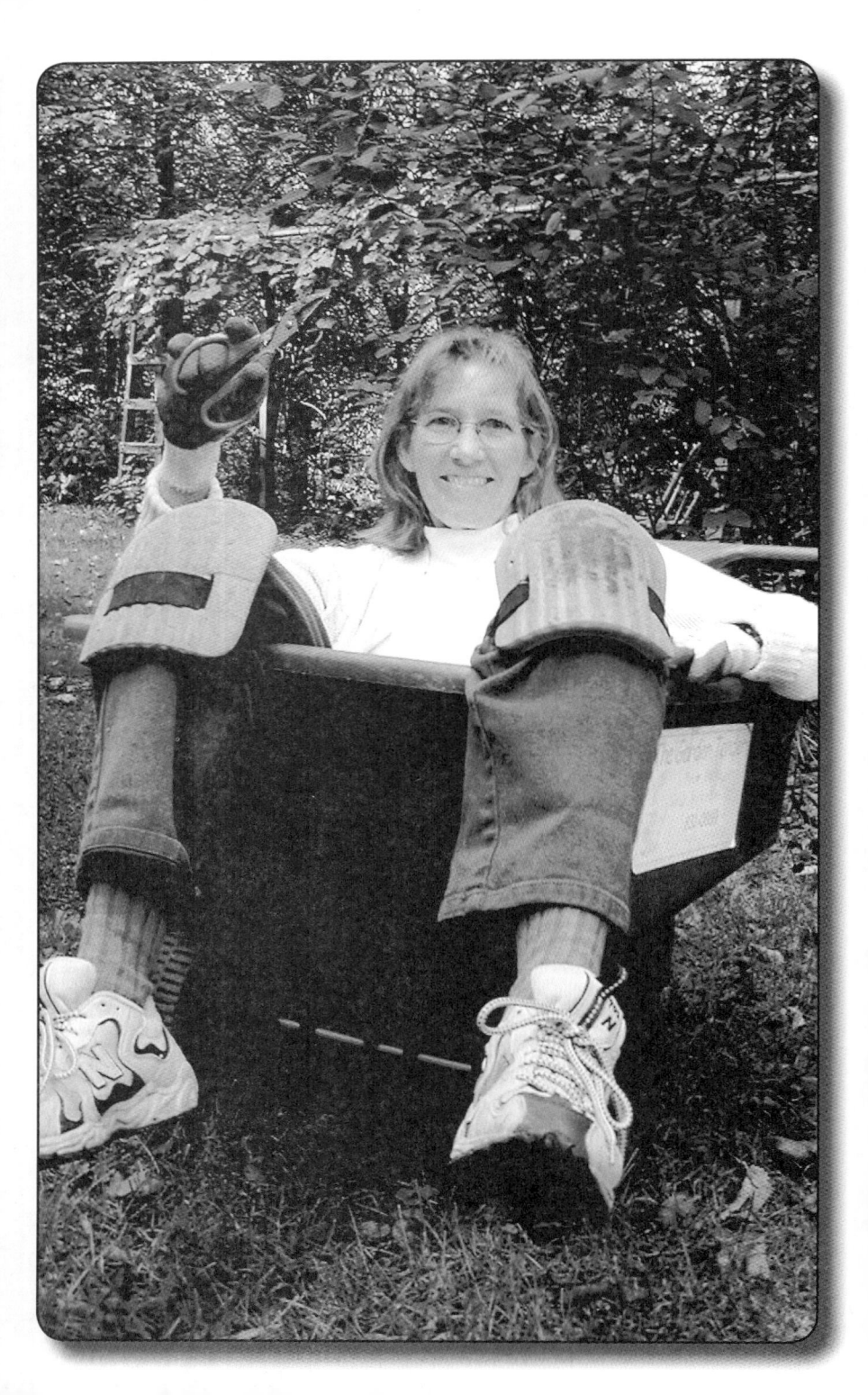

CHAPTER THIRTY
"Kathy! You Did It!"

Dialing 911 set into motion a scene that was every bit as dramatic, intense and chaotic as anything I've ever seen on television. The 911 operator asked several very specific questions about Kathy's situation, then told me to stay on the line and said that she would tell me exactly what to do. First she told me to lay Kathy on the floor, flat on her back. I told her that was a bad idea; that Kathy couldn't swallow and if she was flat on her back she would choke. The operator was quite insistent that I waste no time getting her onto the floor, flat on her back. There was no question that I was no longer in charge. Ann and I moved her from the rocking chair onto the floor.

Next the operator instructed me to tip back Kathy's head and breathe into her mouth. I did. She told me to do it again and then start pressing on her chest over her heart. I took CPR classes eight or 10 years ago, but the instructions the 911 operator gave me didn't match what I was taught. She wanted me to do a lot of chest compressions very quickly, with only a few breaths.

While I was doing this, I saw a pickup truck with the name of a heating company on the door pull into the driveway. *No! You're blocking the way for the ambulance,* I thought. I rushed toward the door to tell him to leave, but before I got there the driver was running to the house with his first responder bag. He was the closest and came right from work.

He quickly checked Kathy's signs. Still no pulse or breath. In one quick motion he cut through her shirt. *You should have worn the clown clothes,* I thought. The responder attached the wires from a small defibrillator to her chest. He adjusted a couple of settings on the defibrillator and I expected him say "clear" and then hear a thunk, like on TV. Instead, the defibrillator spoke, in a woman's voice: "No sine wave detected." I could tell by the man's expression that was not good.

He took the wires back off her chest and told me to once again start the chest compressions. Then he pulled out another device I recognized from TV; a large, clear bulb with a mask attached that is put over the patient's face when the doctor says "Bag him!" Medical dramas were my only point of reference and they helped me understand what was going on.

A moment later, a police car pulled up in front of the house, lights flashing, and stopped in the road just past our driveway. The deputy stayed there until the ambulance arrived a couple minutes later, then he ran into the house, too. While this was happening, I kept the compressions going on Kathy's chest and the first responder kept squeezing the air bag.

The medics quickly checked Kathy's non-existent breath and pulse and told me to pick up the speed of my chest compressions. As soon as the deputy was in the room, they asked him to take over for me. He started doing the chest compressions at the same rate as I was. Too slow, they told him. It should be two beats per second. They set a little flashing light on the floor, next to Kathy's chest, and told him to keep in pace with it. Kathy didn't respond in any way to any of this.

Next the medics put a needle in her arm and gave her a dose of something that got her heart beating again. They connected the needle in her arm to tube and asked Ann to hold the attached drip bag high in the air. As soon as they had a pulse they tried to run an air tube through Kathy's mouth and into her windpipe. They missed. When they pulled the tube back out it was dripping with a thick, greenish liquid that I immediately recognized as the breakfast I'd put into her stomach 30 minutes earlier. They quickly switched back to the bag.

A tanker truck pulled up in front of the house. At first I thought that the squad car was blocking the road and the truck couldn't get through. Then I noticed the driver jump out carrying a medical bag; another first responder.

Anyone who would have driven by at that moment would have been totally confused as to what was going on. Judging by the vehicles on hand—a heating company service truck, a deputy's squad car, an ambulance and a tanker full of heating oil—it probably looked as if we were having an emergency caused by a furnace malfunction.

As soon as the medics felt it was safe to move Kathy, they put her onto the stretcher.

"Where should we take her?" they asked. From the moment that I called 911, the emergency personnel had been in charge, so the question caught me off guard.

"What are my choices?"

They named the two hospitals in town and said that both were the same distance away. That made the choice easy: There was no way I wanted Kathy to wake up in the same hospital where she had her stomach tube surgery. They rolled her through the narrow porch door, breaking off a piece of trim from the desk as they maneuvered around the corner, lifted her into the ambulance and took off, sirens sounding, lights flashing.

The driver of the tanker truck went with Kathy in the ambulance. The pickup driver stayed behind to sort out the medical equipment that was scattered across the floor. I wanted to follow Kathy immediately, but couldn't get out the driveway because of the pickup.

When I finally got to the hospital, I hurried in through the same door they brought Kathy a few minutes earlier and asked where she was. Instead of taking me to her, they ushered me through the ER to the reception desk, where I was asked to fill out some short forms and provide them with insurance information. I asked if I could see Kathy, but was told to wait until someone came to get me.

The someone who came to get me introduced herself as the hospital chaplain. My heart sank. She talked with me for a few minutes, told me that Kathy was still alive, but that she was in very serious condition. Then she walked with me to the emergency room. I took one look at Kathy, connected to a bevy of tubes and wires, and realized that everything she had worked so hard for had been undone in 20 minutes. Even if she survived this day, with all of the drugs and chemicals being pumped into her system, she most assuredly would lose her battle with ALS. I wondered if anyone in the room realized that was the battle she was fighting.

One of the doctors walked me out into the hall. He thought that Kathy had a heart attack, based on blood tests they'd just run. I knew something about blood tests.

One of the tests that Kathy and I had been carefully monitoring, the CPK, showed the degree to which her muscles were deteriorating. We'd been hopefully watching it every four weeks, as it ever-so-slowly dropped from 393 to 351 to 278. The magic number was 140. When Kathy's CPK level dropped below 140, we'd know that she was on her way to winning the battle. I also knew that the CPK test was used to indicate a heart attack.

"Did you do the CPK?" I asked.

"Yes," he said.

"Could you tell me the number?"

"It was 130."

If it is possible to feel both jubilant and heartbroken at the same instant, this was it. She'd made it! God wasn't teasing. Her little steps forward were indicators of what lay ahead. I wanted to run back to her, take her hand and say, "Kathy! You did it!"

Instead I began to cry.

After several stop-and-go hours they moved Kathy into the critical care unit. They did careful studies of her heart and decided that it was strong: The heart attack was ruled out. They did scans of her brain to see if she had a clot from her fall. Everything looked fine. They noticed large spots in her lungs and decided that she had pneumonia. But after going through the entire scenario with me, they decided that, while she definitely did have pneumonia in the hospital, she probably did not have it at home. The pneumonia was most likely caused when breakfast food clinging to the misinserted ventilator tube was blown back into her lungs. In all likelihood, she simply died of exhaustion.

Family and friends arrived and stayed with her late into the night. The kids brought in a CD player so Kathy could listen to a recording she'd made of her favorite songs, hoping that would comfort her. At one point she briefly opened her eyes and we quickly played "Start Me Up." She didn't get up to dance. That was okay. I didn't feel like dancing, either.

The doctor discussed her options. He said that based on the length of time that she wasn't breathing, it was unlikely she could be brought back. If she did regain consciousness, he said she would almost certainly die within a day or two from pneumonia. On the long shot that she survived the pneumonia, he anticipated that she would be on life support for many months. Kathy hated feeling trapped. Our kids, her sisters and I agreed that she needed to be released.

I stayed with her through the night, never letting go of her hand. I'd made a promise to her that I would never leave her alone and I knew she expected me to keep it.

The next morning we all gathered in her room. The life support was turned off. We took her hands and included her in a circle that we formed around the bed.

We said a prayer.

We cried.

We said goodbye.

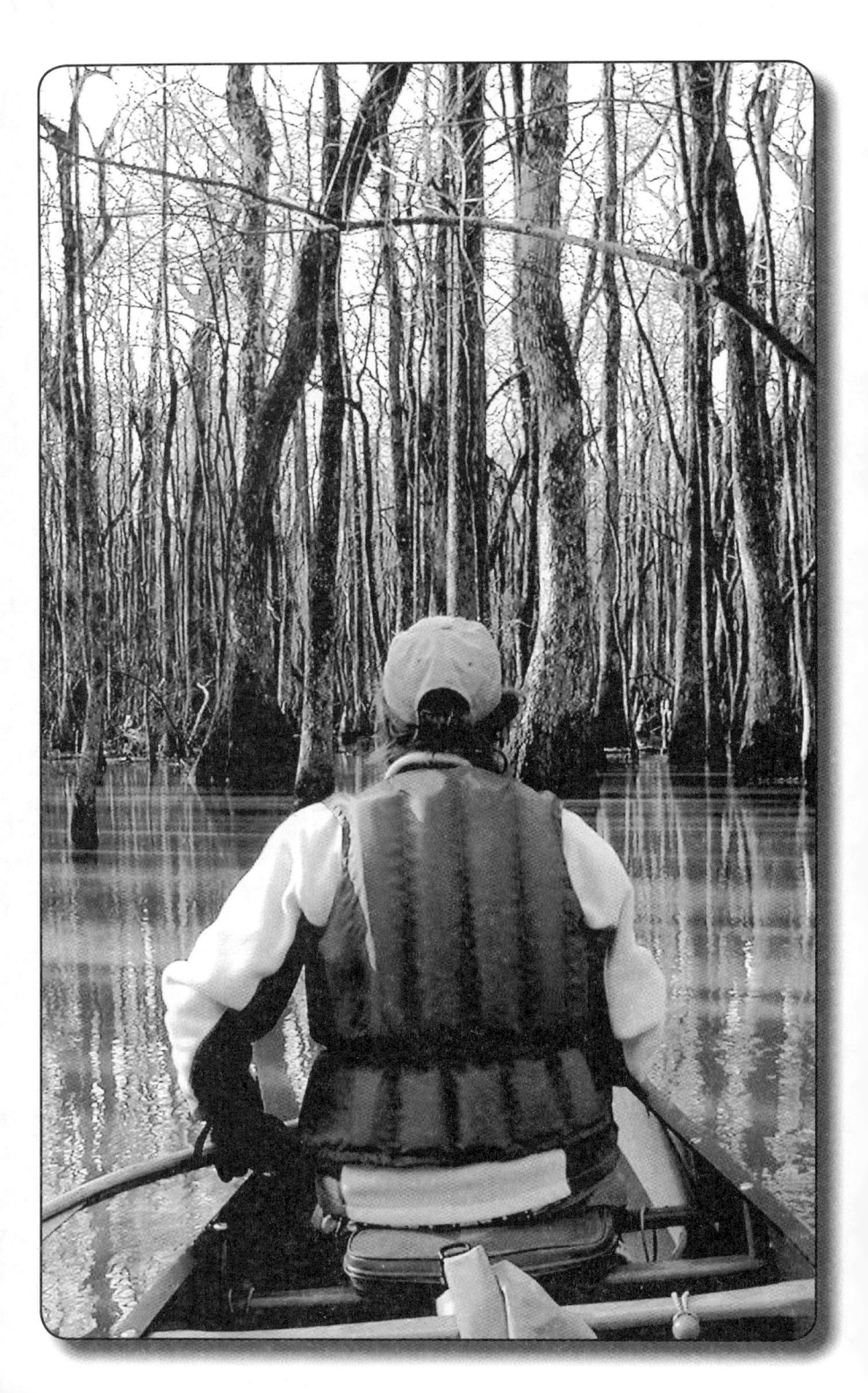

EPILOGUE
The River of Hope

One of the last big adventures that Kathy and I took was in the spring of 2006 when we went to search for the ivory-billed woodpecker in the swamps of Arkansas. It had recently been sighted there after being considered extinct for 40 years. Only one or two people had seen it, though, and its authenticity was questioned. Kathy was determined that we would be the next people to spot it.

After doing some research to know where to look, we hauled our canoe down to the Cache River Wildlife Area, found some locals who helped us get started, and spent a wonderful day maneuvering through terrain that was completely foreign to us. In fact it was foreign to most people, as very few souls had ever ventured into this nearly impassable bayou.

What we discovered was beyond our imagination. We were constantly searching for ways to navigate through the tangle of Cyprus roots and tupelo trees. The path was occasionally marked, thanks to someone who long before us had left a loose series of yellow spots painted on the sides of a few trees. Most of the time, though, we wove our way through and around the barriers completely on our own. Only once did we find solid land, so giving up wasn't an option. We had to see our way through to the end.

After eight hours of careful and skillful paddling, we

came to the end of our quest. We hadn't seen the ivory-billed woodpecker. But we had discovered a whole slough of fascinating and exciting things we'd never seen before.

We had a few scary moments when we wondered if we'd ever find our way out, but each time we managed to move forward together.

After having experienced the elusive bird's habitat, we believed that it easily could have hidden there for 40 years without being detected.

Before we left the area, we bought matching tee-shirts with a picture of the ivory-billed woodpecker above the words "River of Hope."

A year later, on our return trip from Texas, we modified our route so that we could once again pass through the area where we had searched for the hard-to-find woodpecker. Being there again brought back many good memories.

Even though we hadn't found the mysterious bird, we had no regrets for making that earlier journey. We reminisced about it often, shared pictures with family and friends, and told the naysayers that, after having been there ourselves, we believed the elusive bird really did exist.

So it was on my journey with Kathy to discover the elusive secrets that could free her from the monster within her. Unfortunately, we reached the end of our journey before she was healed. But having been there ourselves, we believed that the prospect of healing really does exist.

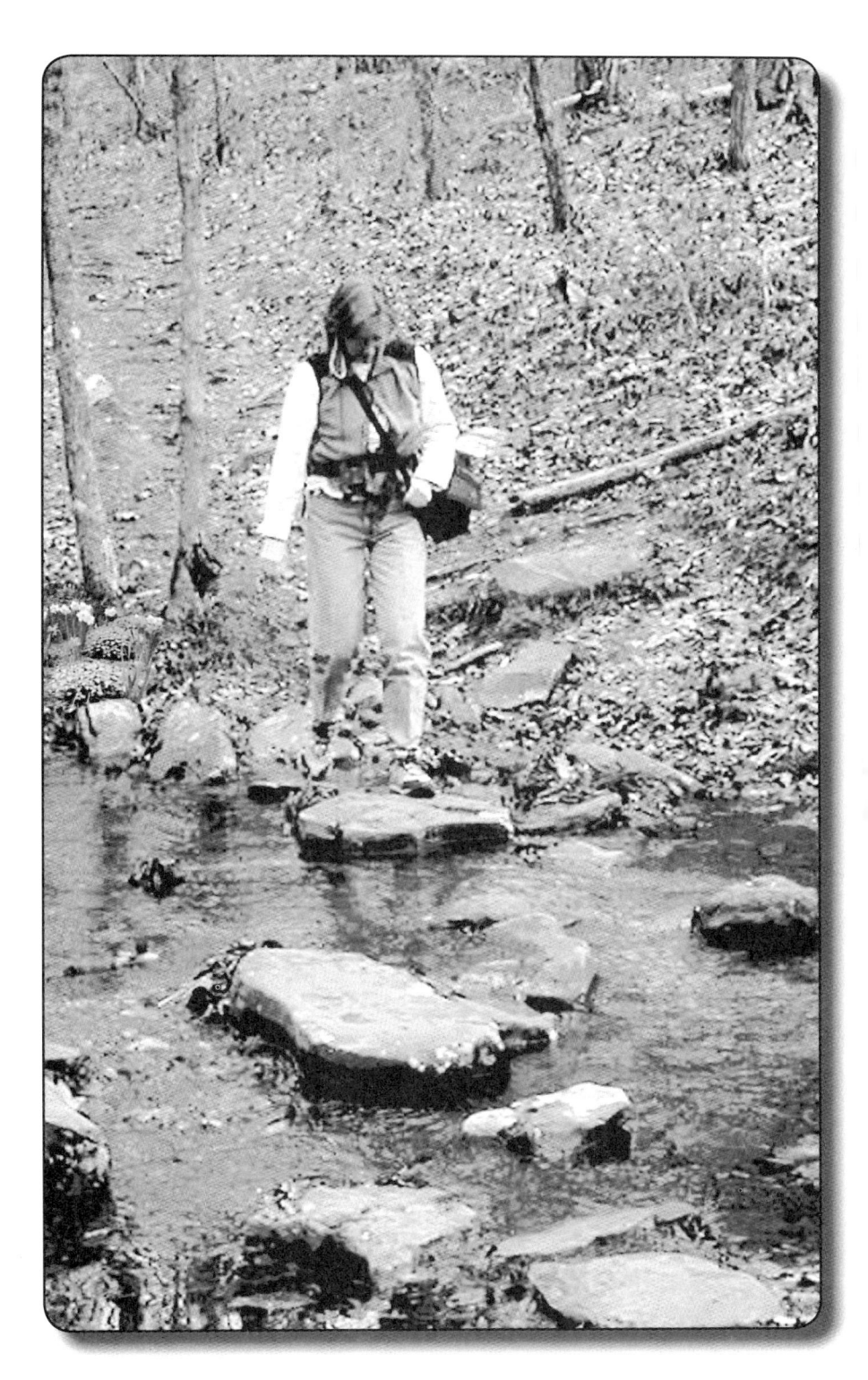